There is beauty in the battle,

Poetry in the perseverance...

If it came easy, what'd be the worth?

So, fight, unwavering –

And pull your dreams to Earth.

-Me

Introduction

My Story

I want to share a bit of my story with you in hopes that it will give you courage to make improvements, however small or large, in your own life. Life's twists and turns often don't make sense as they occur. Sometimes we hit bottom. We find out later that certain events are turning points in our lives. Who survives and who thrives? This can only be answered by the individual. We all have a choice.

Out of my struggles, I found my strength. I found my gift - to help others find their own greatness, harness their own power, and achieve the life they have dreamed of.

In 2008, it looked like I had it all: a career, a house, a boyfriend, a nice car, a close family, and good friends. But I suffered from a near-death experience...of my spirit and soul. My self-esteem was so low that I chose to be in a relationship that ended with trips to the women's shelter and a restraining order. I struggled to make ends meet in a declining real estate market. I spent a few nights without power, because I couldn't afford the bill. I fought with anorexia and bulimia. For a former Division I collegiate track and field athlete, I was out of shape and burned out. It seemed that everything that could go wrong did go wrong, and I was left feeling very sorry for myself.

I needed help. I looked everywhere for answers. I read books, watched videos, and even sought professional advice. No one could help me. I slowly realized that I had my answers – I held the key to the locked door that led to my ideal life! I vowed to change my life into something I wanted to live. In less than two years I went from a broken real estate broker to the best figure athlete in the world. In this book I discuss the methods I used to achieve success, and ways to incorporate them on a daily basis.

Small changes lead to lasting results. Whatever your goals might be, this book can help you hone your strengths to epic proportions.

It's Nice to have an Anchor…or Three

In those dark days, a few things saved my life – my will to fight, my family, and the gym. I vowed that I would not spend another day feeling sorry for myself and punishing myself. My parents offered me a place to stay for a few months after I sold my house. I don't know where I would have lived otherwise! In the gym, I trained with purpose. I would leave feeling stronger – physically and mentally. There was something therapeutic about losing myself in the weights. I found that by conquering the tangible challenge of each workout, the intangible challenges of life became easier to tackle.

I think we all need some type of support system to achieve success and for our overall well-being.

The Big Goal

Through the tough times, I never missed a workout. Training added structure to my day and provided stress relief. I found that I started making healthier food choices and started to feel better about myself. One day at the gym, someone suggested that I try figure competitions. I had always admired the women in the fitness magazines, but wasn't sure about donning a bikini that fits into a Ziploc on stage. I also didn't know the first thing about the tan, posing, hair, make-up, and presentation. But I felt that I needed something – a tangible goal to devote my efforts to.

If You Will It, It Will Happen

When I first stepped on stage, I knew I wanted to take competing as far as I could. I dreamed of winning the Olympia. Many people offered advice as to how I should train, but I decided to train and eat my own way. I wouldn't do excessive cardio or go to extreme means with my diet. I chose to feel good about myself, during competition preparation and during the off-season. I chose balance. I also chose to remain a lifetime natural athlete.

In 2010, I won my first Olympia. I set the goal of winning again – just to prove to myself that it wasn't a fluke. In 2012, I won again.

I proved that it is possible to win the biggest professional figure contest in the world by training smart, eating right most of the time, taking care of yourself, reading, and applying proven scientific methods.

You Are All You Need

In this book, we'll delve into the muscles, the meal planning, and into the mind. We'll start with the mind, as any great accomplishment must be materialized and visualized before it can be actualized. The external tools for success are here. The key factor is you. You hold within you, everything you need in order to excel. I want to share my secrets with you, but I want to also help you discover your own. Greatness exists within all of us, but it's up to each one of us to uncover it and polish it to a shine! Think about your dreams and goals. Consider for a moment that there are no restrictions placed upon you – imagine that you have unlimited resources and time. What would you accomplish? It might seem silly at first, but realize that you have begun to set yourself up for success. Your best life and your happiness are within your reach – it just requires a little stretch to grab it.

Let's get started!

Goals and Success

How Do You Climb a Mountain?

You're standing at the foothills of a mountain you wish to climb. The top of the mountain appears to be unattainable and distant, but despite all of that, you prepare to climb. You stock your bag with a map, tools, and rations. You also have a concrete time frame in mind. In case part of the route is impassable, you have alternate routes. Step by step, you reach the top. As you take in the beautiful view, you stand in amazement when you reflect back on the journey that you experienced while climbing to the top. Setting and achieving a goal is done in much the same way: set your sights on what you wish to accomplish, map a route, create a time frame, gather the necessary tools, and begin climbing step by step. Just like climbing a mountain, you'll face challenges, setbacks, and distractions. But, if you continue making progress, you will reach the top.

In the example of climbing a mountain, the goal is something tangible. I think we're able to cling to a goal much in the same way we'd cling to the side of a mountain. Simply put, set goals you can dig into.

Goals should be in line with your lifestyle. Drastic changes and sacrifices to comfort will usually not produce long-lasting results. For example, if you enjoy living in Florida, your goal of becoming a world-class snow skier would be difficult. This shouldn't deter you from setting large goals, though. If your mind can conceive it, with focus, effort, and patience, you can achieve it. Your mind would never conjure up something that you couldn't accomplish. That concept alone can be scary. Yet, however scary it may seem, continue to cling to it. After a while of thinking this way, you will begin to believe you're capable of pursuing your dreams. More importantly, I hope to help you develop a plan for realizing those dreams.

Requirements for Success

I used to believe that winning a competition meant that I was successful. And in one way, it is. But after the high of winning wore off, I was left feeling empty and unfulfilled. But how could a win not feel like a success? When I set my sights on just winning a show, I wasn't satisfied – win or lose. I went back to the drawing board, so to speak, to assess my feelings and to refocus. I found that the issue exists in the vague and subjective prize at the end of my efforts. To seek approval from 12 strangers (judges) won't bring happiness.

We need more to sink our teeth into. The desire to win helps fuel motivation and pushes us to become better. But concrete goals must accompany this desire. Write down exactly what you wish to achieve by getting on stage. It might be broader shoulders, more developed legs, to improve stage presence or confidence; or it might be to increase exposure for your brand/business. This goes for any contest or subjective setting. Create tangible goals that you will achieve – this way, win or lose, you're a winner by getting up there.

Earl Nightingale defines success as "the progressive realization of a worthy goal or ideal." But what is a worthy goal or ideal? I think it will meet a few key requirements:

- It's objective – something tangible, and something that can be built upon
- It requires a stretch – if it's challenging, it will change us for the better

- It is attainable and in line with your lifestyle
- It's something we really "want" vs. something we think we "should" do

With new a perspective, I redefined my goals. I don't think we ever lose the desire to win, but victories can be achieved on many different levels. For figure competitions, I wrote down specific goals such as building shoulders, adding more shape to my legs, and perfecting my stage presence. I also wrote down specific goals for training such as being able to run 100M repeats at 13 seconds. Career goals came next: one-year plans, and five-year plans. I didn't win my last figure competition, but I met my goals and felt extremely good about it.

The reason I felt so great at the end of that competition was the fact that I met worthy goals that I set for myself. What is a worthy goal? Well, this is something that only you can decide. If you feel that you're challenging yourself and pushing toward something big, chances are, it's a worthy goal. Success isn't just found at the end point of your goal; it is found every day you make progress toward that goal!

Think "Mini" to Maximize Progress

After you have spent some time on your list, break each main goal down into smaller mini-goals. This could be anything from daily steps to monthly steps. The mini-goals serve as checkpoints. It's not possible to climb a mountain with a single step, but it can be done over time. For example, let's say you'd like to work on your running endurance. Perhaps you want to be able to run for 30 minutes straight. Rather than go out and try to run 30 minutes the first time, use that initial run as an opportunity to see how long you can comfortably run before fatigue sets in. Each time you go for a run, add one minute to the time. So, if you run for 10 minutes today, try for 11 minutes next time. I love the idea of non-food rewards for accomplishing pre-determined mini-goals. This can be anything from buying a new pair of running shoes to taking an afternoon off to go to the beach. Give yourself reasonable deadlines for achieving your mini-goals, along with pre-determined rewards.

Setting goals for physique improvements can be done in a similar way. We often make changes millimeters at a time. This is why it's so important to have the main goal in mind, and your mini-goal milestones. We see ourselves every day, so we're often unaware of the changes we're making. This can be discouraging – unless we have methods in place to keep track of our progress.

Tracking Physical Goals

I often talk about living a fit lifestyle and putting the scale away. So many of us use the scale to keep track of progress; but there are better ways. I can think of a time where I weighed in every day. The number on the scale would dictate what kind of day I would have. If I thought it was on the heavy side, I'd be grumpy or more self-conscious. A lighter weight made me feel more confident. If we're not careful, the scale can control us. Toss the scale, and try one of the methods listed below. I haven't been on a scale in months, and have had many more good days because of this.

Pictures are a great way to chart progress. Find a place where you can take pictures every week or every other week. Try to keep the lighting, angles, and outfit the same each time. Also, snap the pictures from the same distance each time. This will help when you go back and compare pictures, side by side. I'm usually not able to fully describe what I have accomplished over time, but can easily show it with the pictures I have kept.

Measurements are another method for charting progress. This can be especially effective if you're looking to gain muscle in certain areas while leaning down. Losing body fat and gaining muscle often creates no change in the scale, which can be frustrating when training toward a goal. Measurements show exactly where the progress is being made. Try to take measurements on a weekly basis, being careful to measure in the same spots each time. Common sites to measure include the calves, thighs, hips, waist, chest, around the shoulders, and the arms. Choose a few areas to measure on a weekly basis.

Another method for tracking progress is calipers. I usually recommend this method if you have someone knowledgeable and reliable to measure for you. When using calipers, measurements can be taken in a number of places on the body. This method of measurement is done with an instrument that pinches the skin (a harmless pinch without pain), and the amount of skin pinched will show how much subcutaneous fat is present at each site. Different people have different methods of pinching the skin – this is why it's key to have the same person track results. I have friends who have purchased calipers and track their own progress, and that's always an option if you want to put some time into learning the basic sites and how much skin to pinch.

Like An Old Friend

Once you have a method for measuring your goals, stick with this method. I have been taking progress pictures for over five years, and can easily compare the pictures to see the changes I've made. But, the same can be done with measurements and calipers. It's possible to make progress quickly, but it can be discouraging to not readily see the results. Not only can the scale be misleading, but so can the mirror. We see ourselves every day and are often not aware of the improvements we're making. Have you ever bumped into an old friend you haven't seen in a while? Have you noticed how she'll comment immediately about any kind of change in your appearance? Since she doesn't see you every day, she can pick up on your progress, even though you don't notice it yourself. Let the forms of measurement be like your old friend — it'll tell you how it is.

I have stressed this before, but patience is necessary. Progress is not a linear journey. Some weeks I'd compare my pictures and not see definitive results, other weeks I would be amazed at the changes. Have faith in your efforts and keep moving toward your goals.

Stay On Track with Support

Surround yourself with a good support system. This can be friends, family, a coach, a fit-friendly forum, or even an app. Accountability is a key factor to staying on track, but it's also nice to know that others around you are striving to achieve their best, too. Lastly, I think it's important to limit the amount of time spent on social media. It can be a great source of inspiration, but it shouldn't be used as a yardstick to measure your own achievements. I have felt my worst when comparing my life to the sugar-coated, filtered, edited lives of people online. Just remember that it's a highlight reel, and you're the real deal.

Remember, the moment you take your first step toward your goal, you're a success. Each step, each rep, each day spent making progress gets you closer to the mountain top.

The Power of Self-Talk

Comparison – The Thief of Joy

"Envy is ignorance, imitation is suicide." Emerson wrote these words, and they seem to hold a deeper meaning. To imitate another is to destroy the unique greatness that lies within you. You are born with a set of skills and gifts that have never before been seen on this earth. Rather than kill your unique greatness, work on honing it and strengthening it. We often wish to have someone else's legs, car, hair, or life. We know our own blooper reel, but assume that everyone else has it better than we do. This is not so! The model's picture on the cover of the magazine is the result of hours of hair and makeup, lighting, angles, Photoshop, spray tanning, and hundreds of takes. She has insecurities, flaws, and even "fat days."

Social media provides another source of false advertising. Scrolling through the news feed, you may see trips to exotic locations, extreme accomplishments, and perfect families. Keep in mind that the image people portray has been groomed, filtered, and carefully constructed – much like the cover of that glossy magazine. Your energy is better spent on yourself, in real life. Stop comparing your bloopers to someone else's highlights. Limit your time scanning through magazines and limit your time on social media.

Maker and Molder

It's called a "work of art" for a reason – the masterpiece you are sculpting takes work!

The artist sits with a lumpy ball of clay. She molds the clay in her hands, encouraging it to take shape. She doesn't lament over the work in progress. Instead, she visualizes the perfect product. Each move of her hands guides the clay into forming the shape she has pictured so many times in her head. The artist is encouraged with each deliberate effort. She touches the form that, until recently, only existed in her mind. After patience and perseverance, the ball of clay becomes a finished work of art. There is beauty in the process – in the entire process, start to finish.

Not long ago, I was cleaning out my storage unit and came across a journal and pictures from college and some time after. I remember always feeling self-conscious. I focused on my bad skin, my frizzy hair, and how I was cursed with inheriting the "Stern shape." In the journal, I wrote about how happy I'd be when I finally "got it together." I was awkward and shy... As I looked at the pictures, I saw myself in a different way. The flaws that plagued my thoughts back then weren't visible now. Instead, I saw my strengths and my beauty. Life happens, and we'll all go through ups and downs, but I realized that the majority of my downs were self-created. Instead of rejoicing in what gifts I possessed, I focused on everything I didn't like about myself. With most of my energy going into beating myself up, it's no wonder why I couldn't wait to be... anywhere else.

In one way or another, we are all artists. However, we don't often take the time to appreciate where we currently are in our personal process. Only by cultivating and sculpting our strengths and forgiving our weaknesses are we able to create a masterpiece.

We All Have Issues

Everyone has body issues. We have hips, "bingo wings," and "big booties." What would you say to your best friend if she ripped your appearance apart? You'd feel hurt, disappointed, your confidence would take a hit, and you'd probably want to smack her. A real friend would never speak to you that way. Yet we allow our inner voice to hiss discouraging words that undermine our confidence and sometimes ruin an entire day.

See Your Strengths

Stop punishing yourself, right now! You are loveable, strong, smart, and beautiful. Look in the mirror and think of the first attribute that comes to mind. It might be your strong legs, your dazzling smile, or even the way you carry yourself. Take a moment and appreciate your strengths, and know they will only improve from this moment forward. It might sound silly, but give yourself a nickname: "Champ," or "Gorgeous" are a couple suggestions.

It's True If You Say It Is

We each have the power to choose our perspective, and thus, create happiness. Sometimes, our perspective could use a little reframing.

How often do you find yourself picking apart your appearance? What's the first thing that comes to mind when you look in the mirror? Take a few moments and write down some negative self-talk or false beliefs you might have about yourself. This is an important step, as we'll work through replacement affirmations below.

With negative thoughts, you might find yourself saying "I can't," or "I'm too __," or "not enough __." If something is repeated often enough, our minds accept it. If you think that you can't get into shape, over time, you will believe it. The false thought becomes reality. Take a look at the negative self-talk phrases you have written down. Cross out each "can't," and replace it with "will." Replace each "I'll try," or "never," with "I am," and "always." Keep each new affirmation in the present tense. Make sure to rephrase the affirmations using positive words, excluding the words "not," or "don't."

Here are a few examples:

- Change "I can't get in shape," to "I will get into the best shape of my life."
- Change "I'm too big/skinny/etc to wear that," to "I will appreciate my curves and strength, and carry myself with confidence."
- Change "I'm too shy to participate," to "I am well-spoken, prepared, and confident."

Again, these are just a few examples, but it will give you the general guidelines for reframing your thoughts. Each time you start to criticize your appearance, stop. On good days, bad days, bloated days, etc., you might find yourself stuck in negative self-talk again. It's ok. Simply take a deep breath and focus on what you like most about yourself. If this is too difficult, try repeating the phrase, "I like myself," over and over again. Bad habits become rooted over time. We may be totally unaware that we're beating ourselves up. It may just come across as a general depressed or foul mood. But, as we start paying attention to this inner dialog, it's important to quickly replace the damaging thoughts with the new, positive affirmations you have created.

This takes time and effort. We build muscles through repetitive exercises, and the brain is no different.

It may seem silly, but dedicate five minutes in the morning and at night to reciting your affirmations. Say them out loud. See how you feel over the course of a week. When you look in the mirror, practice acknowledging your strengths first, and smile! Keep reciting your affirmations, and you will believe them. After all, they're true!

You are beautiful. Not when you have make-up on, not when you lose that last five pounds, not after your morning coffee – right now. Focused repetitions in the gym will create beautiful muscles – focused repetitive positive thoughts will create a beautiful mind. We need both in order to find success.

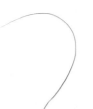

The Fit Lifestyle

Normal?

"I can't wait to get back to normal after my contest." This is a phrase commonly uttered, and at times, I've found myself saying it. Whether it's contest prep, a new meal plan, or even a bikini vacation, we often take temporary drastic measures to obtain our desired results. But, I feel that "normal" isn't always healthy, either. Is it possible to have muscle definition year round and still be able to live the life we want? What is "normal?"

I think we must create a fit lifestyle in order to have our cake and eat it, too. A diet of fast food every other day won't help us look the way we want. But, the occasional cheeseburger can help us stay on track and rev our metabolism. We have the opportunity to create balance – to enjoy a lean physique and the occasional indulgence.

Dieting throws our balance off. But with practice and patience, it's easy to get back. At the very core of this lifestyle is our perception of food and training. Is a chicken breast and rice considered nourishment or a clean meal? If something is seen as a clean meal or diet food, we're more likely to overindulge on junk food later. Why? Well, because we have unknowingly conditioned ourselves to see our meals as a form of deprivation. Instead, look at 90% of the food as nourishment and fuel. We all need protein, fats, and carbohydrate to be healthy and to function.

Cold Fish in Tupperware

Living a fit lifestyle doesn't mean we have to be limited to eating foods out of a Tupperware. Instead, it gives us the freedom to enjoy a treat meal or drinks once a week. It means eating well most of the time, and planning for treats or social events. I used to beat myself up over the occasional Sunday morning pancake breakfast, or buffet with my family. By denying myself what I wanted, I increased my want for more junk food. I would "fall off the wagon" and then tumble for a few days before I could get a handle on myself. Now, I eat without guilt, whether it's a chicken breast and rice, or pizza.

I do keep pre-cooked proteins in my fridge to eat during the week. When I do this, it helps ensure that I don't get overly hungry to the point that I end up eating too much. If you're not a fan of carrying meals with you, know that most grocery stores carry ready-to-eat options like hard-boiled eggs, salad, sushi, and freshly sliced preservative-free lunch meats.

Almost all restaurants can grill chicken or steak. Pair it with a salad and rice, and you have a healthy meal option. I think the key is in making good choices most of the time. Try not to sweat the small stuff. For example, don't worry if the restaurant gave you 4 oz or 6 oz of meat – things have a way of balancing out in the long run.

Human, not Wrong or Bad

Occasionally, we'll slip up and overindulge or have an unplanned treat meal. It's important to acknowledge that we are human – and not wrong, bad, or any other name we call ourselves when we feel badly about what we've done. Enjoy the meal, eat it with mindfulness, and get back to fueling your body the next day. As soon as you start to think negative thoughts, stop them. Remember, you have control over how you think and perceive everything!

Just like dieting can affect how we eat, it also affects our training. Many times, I have added volume to my routine for the last few weeks going into a show, knowing that I couldn't sustain it on an ongoing basis. In order to be as lean as possible on stage, I needed to train twice a day a few days a week. After a contest or shoot, I would struggle to find my equilibrium again. The fit lifestyle is sustainable, and healthy. Realistically, if you can only spend three days a week in the gym, it's ok! Those three training sessions should be intense and meaningful, though. It's also not necessary to have a gym membership. I spent a month traveling with no access to a weight room. Stairs, sprints, jump rope, Tabata circuits, and bodyweight resistance kept me lean and fit into my busy schedule. We'll cover many different ways to train in the next chapters!

Put the Scale Away

When fitness becomes a lifestyle, I think we can toss the scale to the wayside. I used to weigh myself on a daily basis – and the scale would dictate whether or not I had a good day. If I was a few pounds heavier than I thought I should be, I'd put on a flouncy "fat" shirt and frump through the day. If the number on the scale was within my perceived "acceptable" range, I'd leave the house feeling confident. As I write this, I realize how silly it might sound... but I also realize I'm not the only one who thought this way. Let's break things down and look at some of the reasons why these numbers fluctuate:

- Hormonal fluctuations. This can account for a few pounds on any given day, depending on your cycle.
- Lack of sleep
- Hard training sessions and soreness will cause water retention

- Increased carbohydrate intake. For every gram of carbohydrate ingested, the body will hold up to 3 grams of water! This is normal and temporary.
- Increased sodium intake
- Stress
- Overtraining
- Common inflammatory foods (milk, wheat, processed foods, etc)
- Weight will be higher later in the day, after consuming meals
- Adding muscle mass will result in a heavier weight (of course)!

Many things have an effect on our weight. So, if you must weigh in, try to do it weekly. Better yet, try to rely on pictures, measurements, or calipers. Pictures can be compared side-by-side and can offer a dramatic before and after view of your progress. I keep a folder of progress pictures on my computer. When taking pictures, try to keep angles, lighting, distance, and clothing similar from week to week. Measurements will show you actual progress, whether you're looking for broader shoulders or a smaller waist. A tan, a lower-carbohydrate day, and lighting may change the look of a progress picture, whereas measurements are more concrete. Calipers are great for tracking loss of body fat. Areas are "pinched" and recorded. A total of nine sites on the body can be tested (triceps, biceps, shoulder blade, chest, lower back, suprailiac, thigh, and calf). Typically, you'll want to test between 3-5 sites and have the same person "pinch" you each time.

I like having something tangible to compare progress with rather than chasing a number that tells me nothing about my body composition.

Reasons or Excuses

If you have the will, you'll find a way. In 2010, I was living in Ocala, FL. It was a small town, and the people in the gym where I trained didn't understand the sport of figure. I'd mind my business, and quietly train. Every day, either the manager or the staff would make rude comments. I couldn't train elsewhere - it was the only gym in town that had the equipment I needed. I just wore a baseball cap and tried to keep to myself. About three weeks out from the Arnold Classic, I was stopped mid-set by the manager. He said that I was distracting the members of the gym. He asked me to leave, and grabbed my arm to escort me out. I was floored. I couldn't understand why they'd kick me out and make such a scene. As I was pulled outside, I tried to maintain my composure. But once inside my car, I bawled. Where would I train? How could I possibly get ready for the contest without equipment?

I had plenty of excuses to quit – but I had one good reason to keep going. I wanted to win enough money to move to Tampa for a fresh start. I trained in my parents' garage. They had some rusty free weights, a bench, and a giant dinosaur of an all-in-one machine. I sprinted hills, and incorporated isometric body weight training. I didn't care that I had no access to a gym. All I wanted was to place well at the show so that I could move on.

I placed 2nd at the Arnold Classic, and I hit the pavement as soon as the check came. If you have the will, you'll make the way.

What is your reason? The fit lifestyle can be sustained by keeping your goals in mind. What do you want more than anything? Do it. Realize that the path to your goal will never be linear. You will have ups and downs. When I was hit with a setback, I would remember the reasons why I started and remember the reasons why I wanted to achieve that particular goal. If you want it more than anything, you will make a way.

Vampires aren't just in the Movies

When you set a lofty goal, it's normal to feel doubt and experience fear. Protect your goals, and manage your fears. Share your dreams with supportive people and know that there will be many who try to pull you down – especially when you begin making progress. When doubts and fears begin to creep in, remember what you're working toward. Try to surround yourself with people who are moving in the same direction you are – forward. Believe me, it'll make your new lifestyle much easier to attain and maintain. Self-doubt mixed with a partying friend can spell a recipe for derailment. I used to think my crazy friends were spontaneous and fun. However, it's hard to make good choices at 2 a.m. Late nights are fun every once in a while, but it's all about balance. Perhaps meet up with the crazy friend for shopping or lunch instead? This can also be a good indicator as to whether or not that friend is really fun without alcohol.

We can't block out all of the negative people from our lives, but we can limit our time with them. Negative people and "frenemies" will amplify excuses, making it harder for us to create change. Keep your goals and reasons for achieving those goals out in plain sight. It might take the form of a vision board, sticky notes, or it might be a tattered notebook like mine. Choose the method that works for you and don't ever lose sight of it.

Create a Favorable Environment

Just as a plant needs soil, water, and sun to grow, we need a favorable environment to promote the growth we're looking for. Think about ways you can enable yourself to adopt and maintain the fit lifestyle. Here are a few examples of possible small lifestyle changes:

- Buy staple foods in bulk, and cook for a couple of days at a time
- Perfect a few go-to recipes to make eating enjoyable, and also try new recipes/foods
- Install black-out curtains in your bedroom for more restful sleep
- Join an online fitness community like PumpUp to share goals and for overall accountability
- Recite positive affirmations about nourishing your body and using food as fuel (see Self Talk chapter for examples)
- Don't sweat the small stuff. Make good choices most of the time

These are just a few examples. Think about what will help you achieve your goals and create balance. Take a few moments to jot down the adjustments you can make. We reach our goals not with one giant leap, but with a series of small steps. You're setting the stage for long-term success!

Developing the Athlete Mindset

High Octane

A finely-tuned sports car rumbles down the street. The purr of the engine, the shine of its paint – every onlooker recognizes its power. Do you think its owner skimps on fuel, oil changes, and other maintenance? In many ways, the physique is a lot like a sports car. Proper nutrition keeps our engines running on all eight cylinders. We must eat more to burn more. By developing the mindset of an athlete, we're able to eat and train for performance. Our relationship with food becomes healthier and we tend to look forward to training. Each balanced meal and each training session is one step closer to our main goal.

The athlete mindset can be developed and honed by making a few small adjustments over time. The first minor adjustment is to swap out some terminology. Try using the following words, just for one week:

- "Weight room" instead of "gym"
- "Athlete" instead of "gym-goer"
- "Training" instead of "exercising"
- "Perform a set" instead of "do a set"
- "Practice" instead of "session"
- "Re-fuel" instead of "cheat meal"

The words on the left should conjure up different images than the ones on the right. The gym-goer may miss some workouts and drift off track, but the athlete shows up on time and trains with focus.

The idea of performing a set during practice makes the time spent breaking a sweat much more like you're training toward a tangible end goal. And you are. You have your objective goals in mind, and the knowledge that each rep brings you closer to those goals. It's much less tempting to skip a workout or allow someone chatty to interrupt you. Also know that you have someone relying on you to accomplish your goals: YOU!

Food as Fuel

The athlete's mindset can also help us develop a healthy relationship with food. With women especially, we go through periods of "dieting." This can categorize foods as either good or bad. Eating for performance takes some practice, and our mindset can be changed through the use of positive affirmations. "I only eat foods that nourish my body," and "in order to reach my goals, I will eat balanced, healthy meals." A balance of protein, carbohydrate, and fats help to satiate hunger. No food is considered "off-limits" either.

Cravings come and go, but if there's a lingering craving for chocolate or a cheeseburger, plan out an enjoyable meal, one where you can have the exact food you're craving. Set a limit to the treat food, and be present and mindful of each bite. Notice the colors, smells, and tastes of each bite. Savor it. When you're finished eating, that's it – no more food. The next meal should be balanced, healthy, and back on track. No feelings of guilt should surround a planned treat meal. It's a great way to rev your metabolism, and can be something to look forward to.

Drastically limiting carbohydrate or calories can lead to a lower metabolism, and also a decrease in your non-exercise activity thermogenesis (NEAT). This means that the body becomes more sedentary throughout the day, just to compensate for the decrease in calories. This can also cause decreased performance in the weight room. I used to think that I could just cut calories and get to my desired leanness. But, the body doesn't work that way. I would drop a little weight for the first few days, and then the scale wouldn't budge. I was pretty much useless when training, and grumpy and sluggish throughout the rest of the day. Within a few days of increasing my overall caloric intake, I was back to training with intensity and noticed that I was becoming leaner without "starving." Eat more in the form of simple one-ingredient foods, train harder, and burn more.

Reframe Mistakes and Grow

Life happens. Instead of looking at the downside of a missed workout or an unexpected food indulgence as being a fault, know that you're human... and an athlete. The missed workout will allow you extra time to rest and recover, meaning a more intense practice the next time. The overindulgence will give you extra calories to increase the intensity and possibly go for new personal bests.

This mindset takes time to develop, and even after a few years of reframing my mind, I experience times where I'm hard on myself. The difference is that now I can identify when I put on my boxing gloves to try and give myself the ol' one-two punch. I stop the negative thoughts and return to reciting my positive thoughts. In the beginning, it's a good idea to write down a script for yourself. Just like building and shaping muscles takes time and repetition, the thoughts and mind need positive repetition, too! Some examples of positive thoughts, focused on the athlete's mindset include:

- I am dedicated to training
- I am strong
- I am motivated to become the best I can be
- I am powerful
- I am focused on achieving my goals
- I am in control of my own success

You might notice a trend – every affirmation starts with "I am." The "I am" statements are powerful and help us solidify the changes we wish to make. Choose one statement and repeat it ten times. How do you feel? Imagine how you'll feel after practicing this on a daily basis!

Talk To Yourself

I don't think it's a good idea to carry out one-sided conversations with yourself... especially in public. But, practice giving yourself pep talks and focusing on your strengths. Know that if you believe you can accomplish your goals, you will accomplish your goals. A lot of times, our inner dialogue can be detrimental. But, we have control over our thoughts, and can change our thinking patterns to something that suits us better. So, Champ, take a few moments before a big leg workout, or a work presentation to talk yourself into success.

Don't be afraid to dream big. Part of the athlete mindset requires setting lofty goals. If we don't quite reach our goals, chances are, we'll strive for excellence in something else. As a collegiate athlete, I wanted to jump 6' in the high jump. After missing my big goal by 3 centimeters, I dreamed of becoming the best in the world of figure competitions. The drive I learned from dreaming big carries over into everything I do. I know that the same thing will happen for you.

You might find that it's easier to make healthy choices once you adopt the athlete mindset. When training for a goal, proper planning, sleep, and nutrition take a front seat. All of these actions create structure in our lives. Added structure makes us more productive, which in turn helps us to accomplish our goals faster.

Push It

Athletes know that not much is accomplished by breezing through 45 minutes on the elliptical. Much of your training will be challenging, and it takes grit to push through it. Try to push your limits every once in a while. Greater effort yields greater results.

I remember feeling nervous the first time I tried to squat 135 lbs. Even though I had imagined myself performing the exercise, I was unsure if I could really do it. The bar felt so heavy on my traps as I stepped back from the rack. I did three shaky reps, but didn't need help from my spotter. I started to realize that I'm stronger than I believed. We are all stronger than we believe. Strength and success in the weight room equate to strength and success in all other parts of our lives.

Strengthen the Weak

Athletes don't just become successful because of talent, though it can play a part. They show up to practice, every day. When you're working toward something with focus each day, you tend to get pretty good at what you're doing. I think most people miss their workouts because they're mentally tired. When I had my real estate company, I didn't give myself something to train for. I was ok skipping the gym, using lighter weights, and doing part of the workout. I had decided that since I worked long hours, all I needed to do was "break a sweat" in the gym. Of course, I got to a point where I wasn't happy with the way I looked. So, I set out to start training for the high jump again. I rarely missed training days, and pushed myself to get stronger and faster. As a byproduct, I began to like my physique again.

Take a moment to think about your dedication to training. Do you show up to practice almost every day? Do you constantly challenge yourself? If not, perhaps it's time to redefine your goals. Also remember, strength is built in the small decisions and details. Take each training day at a time, push yourself, but be kind.

Repurpose and Redirect Stress

Stress energy can be harnessed into something positive. At its very core, stress is simply a change. Once we're aware of this, it can become easier to choose to look at the change as something positive or as something negative. An injury, for example, is a stressor.

I have broken, torn, and sprained many parts of my body. The first time I broke a bone during training was in college. I ended up having surgery on my foot and was stuck in a walking boot for 6 weeks. I remember feeling like the world was ending because I would have to redshirt. I couldn't train my lower body and came down with pneumonia because I was so upset. Once I stopped feeling sorry for myself, I began to train around my injury in hopes of being able to throw the shot put and javelin. I had always wanted to be a multi-eventer, but never put enough effort into upper body strength training. During my redshirt season, I added 50 lbs to my bench press. Later, I became the first Lady Gator to compete in the indoor pentathlon. My injury turned out to be something good for my athletic career.

I could have saved myself a lot of time and Kleenex boxes if I had just looked at the opportunities that my injury created instead of viewing it as a setback. It was a valuable lesson, and something that I have applied to many of the curveballs that are thrown my way. Mental muscles need the same kind of repetition that our physical muscles need. So, a change in mindset takes careful, focused work. What stress has been thrown your way lately? How can you turn it around into something that will work to your benefit? Take a pen and paper to a quiet place for 30 minutes and write down potential opportunities that the change might hold for you. With practice, this becomes easier over time – similar to the strength we're able to build in the weight room.

Tools for Training

Training Tools

In this chapter, we'll go over some useful tools for creating a training plan, improving overall performance and recovery, and specific physique-enhancing techniques. Topics include free weights vs. machines, benefits of unilateral training, central nervous system and recovery, sprints, and EPOC (exercise excess post-oxygen consumption).

Free Weights vs. Machines

Exercise machines are great for isolation and the development of certain muscles that may be lagging. But if one sticks to training primarily on machines, they end up developing muscle groups separately; resulting in an overall aesthetic that does often tie together well. The use of compound movements through free weights, along with some sport-specific training, are necessary to create a physique with muscle groups that "flow" together.

In addition to developing an aesthetic physique, free weights tend to burn more calories than machines due to the usage of stabilizer muscles that require the body to work harder. I like free weights because of the flexibility in options. For example, if I'm not feeling a certain range of motion, a quick change in hand position or angle will target a different muscle. Sometimes certain exercises can be uncomfortable. Free weights allow me to alter the exercise so that I can train around little injuries or limitations.

Perhaps the greatest benefit to training with free weights is the ability to create endless workouts with minimal equipment. If you're setting up a home gym, a bench and a few sets of dumbbells are a good start!

Machines do serve a purpose, though. If you're just beginning in the gym, machines can be good for learning basic moves and form. I find that they are less intimidating, and most machines display short descriptions and illustrations. Circuit training can be time-saving and will get the heart rate up. Most gyms will have machines set up in a sequence to allow you to work major muscle groups.

If you train by yourself, machines can help you go heavier without needing a spotter. I love the military press machine, as it allows me to focus on the development of my deltoids without worrying about stabilizing the weight.

So, what is the right way to train? Use both according to your training needs and goals! I like to start my training with free weights, and finish with aesthetic/isolation exercises on machines.

Unilateral Training – What is it?

Simply put, unilateral training is any exercise where we train one side at a time. Examples include: single-arm dumbbell row, Bulgarian split squats, and single-leg deadlifts. Training one side at a time allows us to focus more on technique, range of motion, and targeting desired muscle groups.

Symmetry for Stage and Beyond

I realized two things after my first figure competition: no human frame is perfectly symmetric and sports can accentuate the disparity between dominant and non-dominant sides. As a right-footed jumper and a right-armed thrower, my right leg and my right arm were noticeably larger than my left. Determined to improve my look for stage, I spent a few years trying to even out the sides. In addition to unilateral exercises, I would perform drills and jumps evenly on both sides. I worked to build the thickness in my right lat and the width in my left lat to compensate for my ribcage (which is larger on the left side). After incorporating unilateral training, I found that my strength increased in all of my other lifts. I gained speed and aches and pains were minimized!

My story is extreme – you might not have the goal of stepping on stage. But, symmetry is important for a number of different reasons.

Injury Prevention

We're meant to move a certain way. Over time, our routines can cause imbalances. This means that one side of our body might be a little tighter or experience a limit in range of motion. Either side can overcompensate, potentially leading to strains or pulls. Unilateral training is a great way to focus on encouraging both sides to work evenly. When we improve balance, we improve the way we move – in sports, and in general. This means fewer injuries.

Improve Performance and Strength

While performing basic lifts, we may not be aware of the force we exert on either side. When I first started to squat or bench, I didn't care how the weight returned back to the starting position, as long as it went! I think many of us lift that way. One side usually pushes or pulls harder than the other. But, what if we're able to train both sides to bear the same load? Well, we'd get stronger, and perhaps faster! Unilateral training helps us do that. It also helps us become more aware of our body movements, which can also help to improve performance.

Beach muscles

A beautiful byproduct of unilateral training is the ability to improve our aesthetics. Who doesn't love a physique that appears balanced? We've all been to the beach when someone incredibly fit walks by. The first instinct is to stare. The second is to wonder how that person got into such phenomenal shape. Again, if your goal isn't to step on stage – wouldn't it be great to improve appearance? I'll leave it up to you as to whether or not you want to saunter down the beach!

Application

A great way to incorporate the exercises is to swap out traditional bilateral exercises for unilateral exercises. Every exercise doesn't need to be done this way, but perhaps one or two can be utilized per workout. If you're accustomed to benching with the bar, why not try alternating single-arm dumbbell bench press? Swap the squat rack for single-leg leg presses or dumbbell split squats.

For increasing strength and bringing up "lagging" muscle groups, the most effective way is to start the exercise with the non-dominant side, and let it determine the rep range for the dominant side. So, if you're only able to do 6 reps on your left side, do 6 reps on the right. Keep the tempo slow and controlled. This will also help with focus – especially on those last few tough reps.

Visualize and work on the mind-muscle connection. If you can "see" it in your mind, you will be able to see it in the mirror. Target muscle groups by focusing on lifting the weight with just the muscle you're training. Execute evenly on both sides. Often, we'll try to cheat the reps on the weaker side. Be mindful of keeping your body angle the same when executing the set, and pay attention to strict form on reps on the weaker side – limit momentum and bouncing the weights.

I don't think bilateral exercises should be excluded. Just like anything else, balance and variety are great for continuing to see results. While working on bilateral exercises, try to focus on pushing or pulling evenly with both sides.

Train Hard and Recover Well

What is the central nervous system? It's our processing center: the brain and the spinal cord. We tax the CNS anytime we train with heavy weight, especially when we wrap our hands around a bar or dumbbell and make a fist. Stress on the CNS is a good thing in moderation. It's how we cause changes in our physique. "Comfort" and "status quo" usually mean "plateau." But, we must become aware of how much stress we can put our bodies through to make healthy and sustainable changes. I think every person's body recovers at a different rate. In Joseph Muscolino's book, Kinesiology: The Skeletal System and Muscle Function, he states that the CNS can take twice as long to recover than muscles. This is why it's important to listen the body. After a few consecutive lifting sessions, do you ever feel run down? Maybe it's not muscle soreness, but just a general dragging feeling? Many times, this is central nervous system fatigue. Muscle soreness is hard to ignore and easy to identify, but symptoms of a drained CNS can be more difficult to identify. Some of the indicators of CNS fatigue can be:

- lack of motivation
- trouble sleeping
- inability to focus
- getting sick more often

- weights seem heavier than they should
- increased resting heart rate
- plateauing results

Active recovery can be helpful in restoring the CNS. Rather than lifting weights, go for an easy bike ride, walk, or do some dynamic stretching. One of my favorite sayings is "the gym tears and rest repairs." Progress is made while we're at rest. Rest allows us to return to the gym refreshed and motivated!

Incorporating Sprints and HIIT

High intensity interval training, or HIIT, is an effective way to get leaner in less time. But what exactly is it? It's a form of training with periods of maximum or close to maximum effort given to an exercise, followed by a brief recovery period. This is repeated. The duration of a HIIT workout should be between 15-25 minutes. With a warm up and cool down, the total training time will be around 40-50 minutes.

There are many benefits of HIIT training. For one, workouts can be done anywhere: at the gym, track, pool, park, at home – anywhere you have room! You can use equipment, or just rely on bodyweight exercises. Also, the length of the intervals and recovery can be adjusted. Common ratios for effort are 1:2, 1:1, and 2:1. A 1:2 for example, would require more effort, like a 30 second sprint followed by a minute recovery. A 2:1 might be the opposite, where you'd perform increased effort for 2 minutes, followed by a 1 minute recovery.

Some of my favorite workouts are Tabata circuits and sprints at the track. Tabatas are comprised of 4 minutes of circuits – 20 seconds all out, 10 seconds rest. Recent studies have shown that Tabata circuits can burn around 15 calories per minute.

The benefits of HIIT don't stop with time saving! The intense nature of sprints helps to increase our EPOC, or exercise excess post-oxygen consumption. You may have also heard it referred to as the "afterburn."This means that even after the workout is over, calorie burn can be increased from 24-48 hours after.

I like to work in two HIIT or sprint sessions per week, giving myself around 48 hours between sessions. Interval training is much more intense, so it takes the body a little longer to recover than it would with lower intensity training. Try substituting one HIIT workout for your low intensity cardio.

Sample workouts can be found in the Appendix.

A Sprintroduction

As you may know, my background is in track and field. In the time since I ran DI collegiate track, I have continued to incorporate sprints into my routine. I'd often hit up the track until a couple of weeks before competing in IFBB figure competitions.

If you're unfamiliar with sprints, you're probably wondering how to get started. I recommend easing into a sprint routine, both to build a foundation of endurance and to give your body plenty of time to adjust. The goal is to always train without pain, and to never run through an injury. There are plenty of great routines that can be done in the pool, on cardio equipment, or even at home. The pool is great for improving speed, as water has twelve times the resistance as air. Either sprint in chest-deep water or use an Aqua Jogger flotation belt. I prefer the Aqua Jogger because it allows me to fully sprint without touching the bottom of the pool. Yes, it does look silly... but it's effective! Bike sprints should be done at a challenging resistance, while keeping turnover as high as possible. Both bike and pool workouts should last a little longer than outdoor sprints. For example, an outdoor sprint might take 30 seconds. The equivalent on the bike would be closer to one minute to see the same results.

That being said, let's get started! Here are a few tips:

- Choose a soft, level surface to run on. This can be a rubberized track or field. Try to avoid running on pavement, as this will help save your joints.
- Workouts can be "broken" into 100M increments, if you don't have access to a 400M track. This means you'll run a 100M, take a timed break, and run again. A broken 400 is simply 4x100M.
- It's important to build a foundation before sprinting all-out. This can be running a few 200-400m repeats at around 60% of your maximum speed, and building up from there.
- Mechanics are important – swing your elbows through your hips, drive your knees up to parallel, and stay on your toes.
- Spend time on warming up, doing drills, and performing dynamic stretches. Static stretching should be done after the workout.
- From the beginning, keep track of your times. You're looking for a steady improvement – and not to compare yourself to what others are running. If you're challenging yourself, you're getting a great workout.
- A timer watch or GymBoss is helpful for pacing yourself.
- Sprints can be done once or twice a week.

With the transition to the track, the warm up and drills can almost be a workout by itself if done properly. Let's look more closely at why it's so necessary to warm up. A proper warm up will help to increase body temperature, increase muscle elasticity, start the metabolic processes involved with exercise, and to prevent injury. Just like you wouldn't walk out of the locker room at the gym and squat 200 lbs, you don't want to show up at the track and just start sprinting.

After your light 800 meter (twice around the track) jog, you'll want to mark out 20 meters, or about 65' on the track or on the field for sprint drills. You can use just about anything to mark off distance – a water bottle, keys, etc. The focus of these exercises is to take short, very quick steps, but cover very little ground while doing them. Each drill is executed for 20 meters, with a stride/brisk jog out of the drill for about 20 meters. After you have completed the stride drill, walk back to the starting point. Check out my YouTube channel for a quick tutorial and examples of drills! (http://youtu.be/qT6oDhtoDi8 for the direct link)

It will take some time to get used to the warm ups, drills, and workouts. Don't feel badly if you're tired after trying these. If you're still looking to get volume after drills, I recommend running 10 diagonals on the soccer/football field. You'll just start at one corner of the field and stride to the diagonal corner, walking the short side of the field for recovery.

When running on the track, a good initial workout is to run volume at a slower pace. This might mean 2-3x 400 meters, or 2-3 repetitions of one lap. The pace should be around 60% of your maximum effort. This might equate to 20-25 seconds per 100 meters.

Keep track of your times, and gradually decrease the distance while increasing the pace. You can still run longer sprints for sprint endurance, but speed work is helpful, too. A good rule of thumb for sprint endurance is to keep total sprint volume below 1600 meters, or one mile. The total volume for speed work could be anywhere from 400 meters to 1200 meters. The recovery period for sprint endurance can be shorter, usually between 2-4 minutes. Recovery time for more intense sprints should be a little longer – between 4-6 minutes. Don't forget to check out the appendix for specific workouts.

Mind-Muscle Connection

Visualize Your Ideal Physique

Mind-muscle connection is the bridge between visualization and materialization.

You have the opportunity to create the physique you want. You can add muscle, definition, and shape. But you must know what you want before you begin. A sculptor won't pick up a chisel and begin to haphazardly chip away; it's the same as doing exercise after exercise without being mindful. Take a moment and think about your perfect physique. In your mind, "see" the details: strong shoulders, tight waist, shapely legs. This is the first step to developing the mind-muscle connection. Don't worry if you can't imagine your perfect physique just yet. Visualization is just like any other skill in that it takes time to fine tune and develop.

When I first began training for figure competitions, I had no idea of how I wanted to look on stage. I don't otherwise condone comparing yourself to models in magazines, but I found it was helpful to give me a starting point as to what I wished to achieve. Other sources for help with visualizing could be sporting events (track & field, volleyball, etc), or even at your local gym. If you find yourself drawn to the look of certain athletes, it makes sense then to look at how they train. Not only will you be able to begin to see your ideal physique in your mind, but you'll be able to incorporate workouts that will help you achieve it.

Start With Sight

The best way to begin to establish your connection is to work on muscle groups you can see. Biceps, quadriceps, and shoulders are great for this. Let's use the leg extension as an example.

Shorts are a good idea for this exercise. Load the machine with a weight that you can handle easily, maybe 50-60% of what you'd normally do on your first couple of sets. Slowly extend your legs and hold at the midpoint of the exercise. Watch your quads closely and notice how they fire through the rep. You can also place your hands on your quads to feel. Slowly lower the weight and watch how your muscles work. Did you see both legs working evenly? Did you notice your inner or outer quads working harder, or was it fairly uniform? Do another rep and really focus on the movement and the muscle.

Now, turn your toes in slightly, and focus on lifting the weight with just your outer quads or the sought-after "sweep." Slowly raise the weight, see the muscles working...and "see" them working in your mind. With the slower tempo, it's easier to isolate and focus on the details of muscle groups. Slowly lower the weight and focus on just using the outer quads. Again, you can place your hands on your quads to feel where they're firing. Turning the toes out will help you hit the "tear drop" of your quads, but mentally isolating and trying to lift with just that part of your leg will really target it.

Biceps curls are another form of exercise that is useful for practicing mind-muscle connection. Start with dumbbells, and use a weight that you can lift easily. It's easier to focus on the exercise while seated and in front of a mirror. Hold the dumbbells by your side, palms facing up. Slowly curl the dumbbells and continue with palms facing up. Take a second to mentally notice your biceps working. You can also curl one a time, looking down at your muscle or in the mirror. If it helps, put one of the dumbbells down, so you can feel the other biceps working. Think about the muscle fibers in your biceps contracting and releasing. The ability to change grips and angles is much greater with free weights; so this exercise needs more attention and control. Notice the angle of your upper body and know your strengths. Shoulders are often more powerful than biceps, and there's a tendency to lean forward during the set. When this happens, the shoulders start to take on the load, and you won't target the biceps as effectively. Focus on raising and lowering the dumbbells with just your biceps.

It's Not about the Weight

It has been said that the muscles don't know how much weight you're lifting. By slowing down and isolating muscles and details of muscles, it's not possible to do as much weight. But the increased time under tension will make the exercise extremely difficult. That's exactly what you want! Ego has no place in this discipline. There are days for maxing out on weight and hitting personal bests, but those days are helped by increasing your awareness and ability to specifically control your muscles.

"Mirror Muscles" and the Complete Physique

"Mirror muscles" are relatively easy to train. Mind-muscle connection doesn't need to be as strong when we can see the muscles working. I think this is why most of us love to train shoulders, chest, biceps, etc. But one of the keys to a beautiful physique is a well-developed back. Posture is improved, and it makes the waist look smaller. But without mind-muscle connection, it's very easy for the shoulders to do some of the work. One of the best ways to learn how your back works is to invest $5 in a floor-length mirror. Place the mirror in your bathroom, where you can see your back. Watch your back as you squeeze your shoulder blades together. Mimic the motion of a lat pull down, slowly pulling the imaginary weight to your chest. Vary the angles – lean forward and lean back.

Now, try and "flare" your lats. It's a feeling of pushing your shoulder blades to the floor. Close your eyes and visualize how your muscles are working. Open your eyes and check the motion in the mirror. Each time you practice, it'll become easier to "see" how the muscles work, without actually watching them. Take your new skills to the weight room, and practice with light weights. It helps to have a workout partner point out what muscle groups are working, and he/she can lightly touch your lats as you contract them to assist you in feeling them work.

I think that a complete physique can only be built through patient development of the mind-muscle connection. When watching contests, how often does a competitor look like a different person from front pose to back pose? It might seem that imbalances only matter on stage, but they can cause injury. So, a complete physique not only looks aesthetically pleasing, but it can help keep you healthy.

Slow the Tempo

Try slowing down the tempo and becoming mindful of each rep. You won't be able to lift as heavy, but you might find that you'll experience more soreness and achieve a greater sense of awareness with your body and range of motion through exercises. As you advance, try to isolate muscle groups during compound, free-weight lifts. A great example of this is targeting and isolating the glutes during a barbell squat. Studies have shown that advanced lifters have the ability to engage and fire specific muscle groups though the technique of mind-muscle connection. In his study and article, "Mind-Muscle Connection: Fact or BS," Bret Contreras finds that seasoned lifters have the ability to isolate specific muscle groups just by focusing on lifting the weight with those muscle groups.

Mind-muscle connection isn't just for athletes. In a 2004 study by The Lerner Institute, subjects performed 3 months of weight training, with or without visualization. At the end of the study, the group that visualized the muscles contracting gained substantially more strength than the group that didn't visualize.

Lagging or Lazy?

When building a physique, it's very common to have a muscle or group of muscles that are "lagging." Strengthening the mind-muscle connection with those muscles may help to bring up the lagging parts. For example, I had always considered my biceps to be a weaker point in my physique. The truth was, I would often allow my shoulders to take over when my biceps fatigued. After becoming aware of my body, I was able to correct the movements and see results. Another reason for lagging muscle groups is our dislike when it comes to training them. I have found prioritizing my lifts and starting with lagging muscle groups to be an effective way to strengthen the weak points in my physique. If you have a muscle group that you'd like to improve, why not focus on training it when you're fresh and better able to concentrate?

Be Present and Purposeful

What do you think about while you're lifting weights? Are you going through the motions, or are you present, focused, and mindful? Before you work out, take a moment to visualize your ideal physique again. While lifting, continue to visualize that muscle as you'd like it to look. As you get tired toward the end of the set, visualize your target muscles working. Try to eliminate momentum and try not to change angles to make the exercise easier. Be aware of other muscle groups that might be trying to lift the weight for your fatiguing target muscle group. Fantastic physique changes can be made by focusing and pushing through those last few difficult reps. As you train, you'll be able to recognize the burn as your muscles fatigue, and see it as a good thing!

If you're just starting out, I think a workout partner or a trainer would be effective here. A lot of times, we "check out" when we're fatigued. Another set of eyes can help to ensure that the target muscle groups are being worked. With any new skill, practice and patience is necessary. I also recommend taking progress pictures. It's hard enough to notice changes to front of a physique. Comparison photos can also be motivational. We see our bodies every day, and we're often not aware of the changes we've made until photos are placed side-by-side.

Benefits beyond the Gym

One of the benefits of improved mind-muscle connection is the ability to target and sculpt specific muscles. You'll find it gets easier to build muscle in the areas you'd like to build. You also start to notice any inconsistencies from right to left. It becomes easier to fix this.

Perfecting mind-muscle connection also improves awareness, and increases mindfulness in other daily activities. I think that it has helped me be less clumsy. I can enjoy more soreness from the gym, and less soreness from running into things.

Start practicing today, and you'll be on your way to building the physique you've always wanted!

20-20 Training Principle

If I Had All Day to Spend in the Gym...

How often have you thumbed through a magazine and thought, "I could look like that if I had all day to spend in the gym?" Many competitors and models do train for hours a day to achieve their look. This training is usually comprised of lighter weights and steady low intensity long duration cardio. When I first began training for figure, I tried this method. It left me in a time crunch for the rest of the day, caused boredom, and gave me a saggy bottom. I thought that there must be a better way to train.

Being a former collegiate athlete, I still loved the ability to train for strength, speed, and power. I wanted to be able to sprint a 100M in 13 seconds on any day, squat my body weight for reps, and jump up on the tallest plyometric box. This translates into other activities, such as carrying all of the groceries into the house in one trip, and climbing 5 floors of stairs without being winded. I think it's important for all of us to have something we want to get stronger, quicker, or better for.

In addition to being functionally fit, I wanted the ability to have more control over how my physique looked. I have always been drawn to the aesthetics: the sweep of the quad, the cap of the shoulder, or the peak of a well-built biceps. I found that training for function helped with aesthetics somewhat, but it didn't quite improve the finer details.

This all brings me to my next question. Is it possible to have the best of both? After years of experimenting with different training styles, I came up with a method that allows for improving athleticism and aesthetics: The 20-20 Training Principle.

The basis is fairly simple, and can be adjusted to fit your goals. For the first 20 minutes of training, you'll focus on compound exercises that build strength, power, and maximize calorie burn. For the second 20 minutes of training, you'll focus on isolation exercises to sculpt specific muscles. I noticed that I didn't need traditional cardio, and I was able to maintain a lean physique year round. The only drawback - the workouts are challenging!

Let's go over the specifics and look at ways to tailor the training to fit your goals.

The First 20: Sport, Strength, Power

Sport-specific training includes a variety of compound movements which have many benefits. Compound movements are multi-joint exercises where you'll use two or more muscle groups. This training relies mostly on free weights. The use of free weights can encourage a more natural range of motion, improves balance, and engages stabilizers. Not only does this make us stronger, but it helps us burn more calories in less time. I rely heavily on the six basic compound lifts. I have listed them here, along with just a few variations.

- Squats (front, back, split, hack, lunge, goblet, sumo)
- Row (barbell, dumbbell, t-bar, wide-grip, Pendlay)
- Bench press (barbell, dumbbells, flat, incline, decline, close-grip)
- Pull up/chin up (wide, close-grip, plank, single-arm assisted)
- Overhead press (barbell, dumbbells, Smith machine, wide, unilateral)
- Deadlift (single-leg, sumo, elevated, straight-leg)

Listed in parentheses are just a few of the hundreds of variations that can be created from these lifts. In addition to weights, you can incorporate Olympic lifts and plyometrics. Both are a great way to practice explosiveness and get the heart rate up. I also find that I perform better if I start my training with challenging, compound exercises while I'm "fresh."

Usually, I fatigue after about 20 minutes of intense training (either muscles or central nervous system). This is a good time to switch gears and focus more on sculpting muscle groups.

The Second 20: Sculpt

Since isolation movements are much less taxing, they tend to work well at the end of a workout. Isolation movements are also great for working on aesthetics. Isolation movements are single-joint exercises where one muscle is being worked. Some examples include:

- Biceps curls
- Leg extensions
- Triceps extensions
- Front delt raises

Isolation exercises can be made more effective and challenging by lifting the weight with both legs, and performing the negative with just one leg (alternating each rep). Lighter weight must be used for this, but it's a good way to build strength and break through plateaus. You may choose different exercises, depending on your goals and resources. If you need more hamstring work, choose two hamstring exercises for the isolation supersets.

If form is an issue, you can opt to use more machines during this time of training. Machines are great for targeting specific areas of a muscle. They also allow us to train without heavily engaging stabilizers.

Since the main focus is on sculpting during the last 20 minutes of training, stay present and mindful with each rep – whether you're using free weights or machines. This can take practice, as we all have a tendency to "tune out" when we start to fatigue. Remember that the greatest physique improvements often happen during those last few difficult reps.

Tempo for Recovery and Repetitions

In college, the recovery time between sets was usually between 2-5 minutes, depending on the lift. We usually had an hour or two to do just a few lifts. But, I have found that a shorter recovery period will keep the heart rate up while saving time. Aim for a recovery time that ranges between 45 seconds to one minute between your sets. If you keep an eye on your watch, you'll notice it's not a lot of time.

The pace of each repetition will depend on your goals. I have found that a slower lifting tempo will help with gaining and shaping muscle. For this method, a set should take between 45 seconds to a minute to complete. While 45 seconds for recovery is not a lot of time, it can seem like an eternity during a training set.

I also like performing the concentric part of the exercise at a regular pace, and drastically slowing down the eccentric (negative) part of the exercise. I think this helps increase strength and can help to sculpt the muscle.

In training for power, the tempo is usually faster. Repetitions are performed as quickly as possible. Hang cleans, jerks, and plyometrics are a great example of this.

For general lifting, a tempo that's slow enough to engage the mind-muscle connection is good. Changing the tempo of the workout can be enough to break through plateaus. So, don't be afraid to experiment with faster or slower reps, and adjusting the recovery time between sets.

Choosing Set and Rep Range

The number of sets and reps will depend on your goals – you can choose light weight and high reps with a short recovery time, and this will act as more of a cardio workout. So, if your main focus is to lean down, you might try incorporating circuits, giant sets, and supersets of compound movements. An example of a giant set might be:

- 3x15 dumbbell shoulder press, upright rows, and push ups – exercises performed back-to-back with 30 seconds recovery between giant sets.

Or, you can focus on lower reps with heavier weight to work on strength and power. I love pyramid sets for strength. An example is:

- 10/8/6/4 reps of squats, increasing the weight each set.

In the times where I wanted to add muscle, 4-5 sets of 8-10 reps were effective for me. I feel that increasing the volume of training will help with hypertrophy. I tend to prefer straight sets for gaining muscle, as it allows me to focus on one muscle group (or one specific area). I think weight should be challenging for the last few reps, but not so challenging that form is sacrificed.

The greatest physique changes seem to be made during those last few tough reps. Proper form and being mindful is so important. An example of a hypertrophy set is:

- 5x8 squats, pause below parallel, and take one minute recovery between sets.

Remember, the body is amazingly adaptive. A particular set and rep range may be effective for some time, but it's a good idea to incorporate different techniques into your program. This not only prevents a plateau, but it can also prevent boredom.

Training Splits

If you have 4 days to train per week, try doing two upper body days and two lower body days. I like setting up push-pull workouts in supersets, as it gives the opposing muscle group time to recover, keeps the heart rate up, and maximizes time spent in the gym. On a 3 day split, try one total body day, one upper body day, and one lower body day. Even if you're not in a time crunch, it can be an effective way to break through a plateau with your current training.

Sample Training Day

This style of training can be applied to any training day, from a heavy leg day to a push-pull workout. For example, on a leg day, the exercises might look like this:

- 5-10 min warm-up with dynamic stretches
- 3-5x5 sets of hang cleans
- 3x8 squats superset with dynamic bench step ups (8 each leg)
- 3x8 hack squats superset with dumbbell Romanian Deadlifts

- 3x8 leg curls superset with leg extensions
- 3x10 sets of hip thrusts superset with calf raises
- Additional isolation work, or cool down and stretch

The exercises in each superset should be performed back to back. It's important to use strict form, keep the reps slow and controlled, use challenging weight, and to be smart about training. There are times when I want to go heavier on squats, but I don't have a spot. In this case, I'll either increase the time under tension on lighter weight by pausing 2-3 seconds at the bottom of the rep, or I'll go heavy on leg press.

Arm Day

Many of us end up with an "arm day" for training. When I started competing in figure, I would train arms in the traditional way of bodybuilding: countless isolation exercises. I found that this wasn't maximizing my time in the weight room, and that this type of training didn't help me get leaner. So, I started using the 20-20 Training Principle for arm day. Here's an example of what one of my workouts would look like:

- 5-10 minute warm up with dynamic stretches
- 4x10 close-grip bench
- 4x10 plank chin-ups (focus on pulling with biceps
- 4x10 weighted bench dips superset with single-arm assisted pulls
- 3x10 skullcrushers superset with standing hammer curls
- 3x10 triceps extension on cable superset with drag curls on cable

As you can see, it's possible to incorporate compound movements into an arm day workout. Again, this helps to increase overall calorie burn and it saves time. I also like the fact that it allows us to work chest and back. This can help loosen tight muscles and allows us to see results more quickly.

For more training ideas and specific workouts, check out the appendix.

Creating Your Training Plan

Let's Train

In a previous chapter, we discussed the difference between exercising and training. Exercising can be compared to getting into your car and just going for a drive - you may end up reaching your destination, but you'll more likely end up burning gas and time. Exercising is great for someone who is just looking to maintain a certain physique, and it's certainly better than nothing. However, I have found that it lacks challenge, which is a key factor to staying motivated and engaged. Transitioning from exercising to training is a great way to create challenge. When you approach your workouts with the focus of training for something specific, you'll find less distractions and more motivation. By working toward objective goals, you'll develop the habits of an athlete: more drive, focus, and dedication!

Let's take a look at the goals that you have established. First of all, you must identify your goals. What is your primary goal? Do you wish to work on muscle definition, strength, or are your goals more related to improving endurance? Next, think of 1-2 other goals that are important to you. At this point, I would recommend a total of 2-3 goals. It's also a good idea to make sure these goals can realistically be achieved at the same time. For example, it is possible to gain muscle and lose fat, but not as possible to gain muscle and train for a full marathon?

Identifying your primary goal will help you with assigning order to your exercises. Most training sessions should begin with exercises that will help you achieve your main goal. If you really want to win your next 5K or Spartan Race, work on your endurance or cardio first. If your goals are strength or physique-related, hit the weights first. If you just wish to be leaner, perhaps a mix of weights and cardio would work for you.

Define Your Schedule

How much time can you devote to training? You might work from home and have all the time in the day to train, or you might have a full time job with a family and only 30 minutes to train. Be realistic about this part. If you only have 30 minutes, that's fine. There are many ways to structure a plan that will still allow you to see great results.

How many days per week can you train? This will help you design your training split. Training splits can be as dynamic as your schedule. In the 20-20 Training Principle chapter, we went over how to plan your set and rep range based on goals. In this chapter, we'll cover how to put that information into a plan that will work for you – whether you train 3 days a week or 6 days a week. After a while on one split, you might decide to change to another. Let's take a look at some options.

Training Splits - 3 Days Per Week

It's possible to make improvements in strength and physique on a 3-day training split, but the time must be used effectively. I would choose mostly compound movements to get more "bang for your buck," as the isolation/detail lifts tend to be time-consuming. Depending on your goals, training can be divided accordingly:

1. *Total Body:* Each day you'll work on legs and upper body. This can be done in straight sets or supersets.

Alternate a leg exercise with an upper body exercise in a superset to keep your heart rate up while allowing the other muscle group to rest. An example of a superset might be a squat with a military press.

2. *Legs/Upper Push-Pull/Total Body:* Here, you'll focus on one day dedicated to leg training, one day of upper body push-pull, and one day of total body training. This split allows for more recovery time between lifts. Push-pull exercises also allow the antagonist/opposing muscle group to rest. For example, you might try pairing bench press with a dumbbell row.

3. *Hybrid:* You may decide on an upper body day, a lower body day, and a conditioning day. Some lifters would rather train legs once a week, and divide upper body into two days. Again, this will depend on your goals. See the appendix for a sample 3-day building program.

Training Splits – 4 Days Per Week

A 4-day split allows for a little more flexibility and time to focus on detail work. An easy option for planning would be to take a 3-day split and add in a cardio or conditioning day. If you'd rather lift, check out these options:

1. *Upper-Lower:* You'll train upper body twice a week and lower body twice a week. Train four days in a row, or complete two lifting days, take a day off, and complete the next two days. The splits can be organized into distinct muscle groups. This can either be push-pull or muscle group specific. So, you might do chest and back one day, and shoulders and arms for the second upper-body day. Legs can be worked in the same manner.

2. *Push-Pull:* Here you'll train muscle groups that push one day (chest, legs, shoulders, and abs) and pull another day (hamstrings, lats, and biceps).
3. *Major Muscle Group with Isolation Work:* This split allows for more physique building. You might do chest, shoulders, and triceps one day, back and biceps another day, and legs twice a week with one day focusing on quads and calves and another focusing on hamstrings and glutes.
4. *Hybrid:* You may decide on an upper body day, a lower body day, a total body day, and a conditioning day. Or, you may choose part of a regular 4 day split and swap a conditioning or cardio day for one of the weight days. In college, we were typically on a 4-day split – 3 days of strength and power training with one day of upper body maintenance. Your goals should dictate what you spend most of your time on.

Training Splits – 5 Days Per Week

A 5-day split allows for a lot of flexibility in planning. Training days can be Monday through Friday, or can be in a 2 days on, one day off format. This split is also great for an athlete who is looking to perfect skill-work, aesthetics, or work on mileage. Here are a few options for scheduling the days:

1. *Upper-Lower with HIIT:* You'll train upper body twice, lower body twice, and do conditioning/HIIT training once. You can also perform an additional HIIT circuit after one of the upper body training days.
2. *Push-Pull with HIIT or Conditioning:* Two days of training muscles that push, two days of training muscles that pull, and one conditioning day.

3. *Major Muscle Groups:* Chest, back, legs, shoulders, and arms have a designated day. This is a good split for building muscle. Conditioning can be added to the easier upper body days.

4. *Hybrid:* Any of the splits can be adjusted, depending on your goals. For example, if the goal is to build legs, they can be trained twice a week. Simply combine upper body muscle groups (either push-pull or a major muscle group with isolation work). If the goal is strength and power, there might be three days of lower body training with a day of HIIT/upper body maintenance, and a day of skill work or active recovery.

Training Split – 6 Days Per Week

This split should take recovery (CNS and physically) into consideration. I think it's important to monitor the intensity of a 6-day split. One or two of the days should be higher volume, lower weight, or active recovery days. I would typically use this split when preparing for a contest or during times that I knew I could get proper nutrition and rest. A 6-day split allows for almost unlimited options for planning. Let's look at some:

1. *Body part split with emphasis:* Each major muscle group has its own day, with an additional day for bringing up a lagging muscle group. If the goal is to build shoulders, training frequency can be increased to twice a week.

2. *Push-pull with conditioning or skill work:* This is similar to the 4-day split, but allows for two days of focus on skill work or conditioning. This is also good for mileage training or speed work where two days of the week can be spent by doing road work or a workout at the track.

3. *Major muscle group with isolation and emphasis:* Back and biceps, chest and triceps, shoulders, and legs will

each have a designated day. The lagging muscle group can be worked on the sixth training day.

4. *Hybrid:* More training days mean more options. Again, look at the main goals to determine splits. You might want to run a marathon. If so, three days of total body strength training with three days of road work might be a good split.

Slippers are Comfortable, Training Routines Shouldn't Be

The human body is amazingly adaptive. After a certain time of going through the same routines in the weight room, it adjusts and becomes more efficient at getting the job done. In many other situations, efficiency is to our benefit. But, when it comes to the expectation of continued physical progress, efficiency can cause us to plateau. This is why I recommend adjusting your training as soon as it becomes comfortable. "Comfortable" often means "plateau."

There are many ways to break through a plateau. It doesn't always require a complete overhaul of your training. Here are some tips that have helped me along the way:

- change the muscle groups worked/splits
- switch from straight sets to supersets or circuits and vice versa
- change the order of your exercises (pre-exhaust)
- change grips or stances
- switch bilateral exercises for unilateral exercises
- change the number of sets/reps (from 4x8 to 5x5, for example)
- decrease recovery time between sets
- increase the amount lifted each week
- change up your goals
- get a workout buddy

- try a new class
- take it outside, to the pool, the park, etc
- get new workout music
- read up on different training disciplines
- change the order of your exercises (pre-exhausting muscles, for example)
- If you do cardio, vary machines and interval and rest periods

Tools for Meal Planning

Researching Ratios

When planning my meals, I stay around a 40/40/20 ratio: 40% protein, 40% carbohydrate, and 20% fats. Depending on my level of physical activity, I keep my calorie intake between 12 and 16 calories per pound of bodyweight. For example, a 140 pound woman would eat between 1,680 and 2,240 calories per day. I feel that most meal plans will be effective; it's just a matter of finding one that fits your needs and lifestyle.

I have a few guidelines that I tend to follow regarding the meal timing of carbohydrate and fats:

- When I'm not training in the morning, I eat a combination of protein and good fats. An example of this might be 4 egg whites, one whole egg, and half of an avocado. Research has shown that starting the day with protein and fats helps us utilize more fat for energy throughout the day.

- I tend to eat most of my carbohydrates around training times; about an hour and half before training, I'll have around 30 grams of carbohydrates, 30 grams of protein, and a small amount of fats. An example might be 4 ounces of chicken and half of a cup of brown rice. I'll have 30 to 40 grams of quick-digesting carbohydrate and 30 grams of protein after a workout. An example would be an apple and a whey protein isolate shake.

- The body is most anabolic post-workout. This means that if we choose to eat extra calories, it should be done within an hour or so of training. I would recommend trying different macro combinations after training in order to see what your body responds best to.

- Calorie intake, especially carbohydrate intake, can be increased on days when larger muscle groups are trained. Leg workouts, back workouts, and days with plenty of compound movements can all be higher carbohydrate days.

Turn Up the Volume

If I'm very hungry and choose to increase the size of my meal, I'll increase the amount of protein. It's very difficult for the body to convert protein to body fat. Protein also has a satiating effect. We feel less hungry when we eat more protein. I also don't weigh my proteins, unless I'm two or less weeks out from a competition. This helps me to eat according to how I feel at the time.

Vegetables, for the most part, are considered "free." I fill up my plate with brightly colored veggies and richly spiced healthy foods. Just like the old saying, "we eat with our eyes first," if the plate is sparse, we'll feel like we haven't had enough food. Don't underestimate the visual appeal of a full plate or bowl. Sometimes, I'll put an entire bag of spinach in a large salad bowl. I'll throw some rice and chicken on top, and that will be my meal! It's usually around 300 calories, but looks like a mountain of food! Increased protein intake, along with increased volume of foods leads to satiety.

One of my favorite books is *Volumetrics*, by Dr. Barbara Roll. In the book, Dr. Roll theorizes that the body is accustomed to eating a certain volume of food. We can either eat that volume in high-calorie, nutrient-poor foods, or in low-calorie, nutrient-rich foods. Which one of the following would you rather eat?

Would you prefer a greasy drive-thru burger or grilled steak, a baked potato, steamed veggies, and an apple?

What Works for You

I think we all need to eat simpler, one-ingredient, whole foods. But I think it's even more important to find a macronutrient split that we can live with. I saw great results in my physique when I switched to a low-carbohydrate, high-fat diet, but I just couldn't think straight or perform well during intense training. I think that any macronutrient combination that's based on moderate caloric intake can be effective. But, we should be able to function and feel good.

A rule of thumb that I have used in the past is to think about the types of food you might crave when hungry. Is it a sugary, crunchy food? Or do you crave comfort foods that are very rich? Chances are, if you crave richer foods, a lower-carbohydrate eating style might be a better fit. I have plenty of friends who live on steak, almonds, and avocados, and they maintain a healthy weight year round.

We each have different tastes, preferences, and activity levels. It can take some time to find an eating style or styles that work best. It might be a hybrid that you design after a few weeks of trial and error. Whatever it might be, the following calculations should help provide some guidelines.

Quick Calculations

As much you might want to reach your goals quickly, drastically reducing overall caloric intake tends to be more harm than help.

Some quick calculations will help you find your Basal Metabolic Rate (BMR), or the amount of calories your body needs on a daily basis just to survive. Most of us do more than lie in bed all day, so we'll need calories in addition to the BMR caloric intake. The best resource that I have found for calculating BMR is bmi-calculator.net. Once you know your BMR, some quick calculations using the Harris Benedict Formula will help you find what your target caloric intake should be.

To determine your total daily calorie needs, multiply your BMR by the appropriate activity factor, as follows:

- If you are sedentary (little or no exercise) : Calorie-Calculation = BMR x 1.2
- If you are lightly active (light exercise/sports 1-3 days/week) : Calorie-Calculation = BMR x 1.375

- If you are moderately active (moderate exercise/sports 3-5 days/week) : Calorie-Calculation = BMR x 1.55

- If you are very active (hard exercise/sports 6-7 days a week) : Calorie-Calculation = BMR x 1.725

- If you are extra active (very hard exercise/sports & physical job or 2x training) : Calorie-Calculation = BMR x 1.9

If your goal is to get leaner, you can subtract 200-300 calories from your result. This will give you a caloric deficit without sending your body into starvation mode. Again, when your training volume or intensity is increased, you can increase your caloric intake, especially post-workout.

Tracking Macros

Generally speaking, if you're concerned with maintaining a certain weight, watching overall macronutrient intake could be effective for you. But, if you're concerned with body composition, paying attention to the quality of protein, carbohydrate, and fats will help you move closer to your goals. You will probably see genetically gifted people noshing on nachos and ice cream, all while maintaining six-pack abs. Most of us aren't able to eat that way every day and stay lean.

I don't think that all calories are created equally. Pop tarts and a protein bar might have the same macronutrient breakdown as a chicken breast, sliced avocado, and an apple. However, the quality of calories will vary greatly. The body will easily assimilate the protein from a chicken breast, but probably won't be able to utilize all of the protein from a bar. Bars tend to contain collagen, soy, and other protein sources that contribute to the overall protein grams – but won't help to build or maintain muscle like a whole food will. Preservatives, food colorings, and additives also make the pop tart and bar harder to digest.

To sum it up, I think tracking macronutrients can be a fun and flexible way to maintain a certain weight and take the monotony out of a meal plan. But, for overall long term health and body composition, simple one-ingredient meals can't be beat. I also think it doesn't need to be one or the other. In fact, I would recommend trying different eating styles to see how your body reacts.

Carbohydrate Cycling

A simple fix is to continue to make progress it to make sure calories never drop below the Basal Metabolic Rate (BMR). Also, I think it's important to eat frequent, balanced meals. If you must restrict calories, try carbohydrate cycling. A simple way to jump start your way to leaning down is to go low carbohydrate and low calorie two days a week. This should be done on days off from the gym or on easy low intensity days. You'll keep protein intake the same, and drop carbohydrate intake to between 30 to 50 grams for the entire day. If you're working out that day, carbohydrate intake should occur before and after your training, Two days a week is enough to help you see results, to be bearable, and to prevent your metabolism from slowing down.

The Liver and Metabolizing Fat

The liver has many functions; from detoxifying the blood to helping to metabolize fat. It's basically a filter for our bodies. When we have the goal of leaning down, I think it's important to make the liver's job as easy as possible. When we streamline our meals by eating simple, one-ingredient, fresh foods, we allow the liver to work more on metabolizing fat. If we consume artificial sweeteners and processed foods, the liver must work harder to break down these toxins and won't be as efficient in metabolizing fats.

This process can be likened to a water pitcher filter. When a few teaspoons of sand are tossed in the filter, it still manages to function efficiently. Now, imagine dumping a few cups of sand in the filter. The water flow may turn into a trickle, and the filter has more of a difficult time producing clean water.

Try to keep artificial sweeteners and processed foods to a minimum for two weeks. Without changing anything else in your meal plan or training, I'll bet you see results!

Assessing Food Allergies

It's important to be aware of food intolerances. Certain intolerances could possibly be the cause of delayed progress and reduced performance. Though there are several tests for allergies and intolerances, no one test has been shown to be fully effective. You may wish to speak to your doctor. In addition to going to your doctor, a few weeks can be set aside for an elimination diet to see if you feel differently.

After doing some research, I decided to eliminate common inflammatory foods from my diet for two weeks. These foods include: wheat, dairy, sugar, peanuts, and processed foods. This also forced me to read labels. I found that many boxed products contained added chemicals and wheat products. After a few days of simple, one-ingredient, whole foods, I began to have more energy. I also started to lose size from my abdominal area, and no longer had a runny nose. It's amazing to realize how many bothersome little issues we live with on a daily basis. What's more amazing is the fact of how these issues can easily be cured by eating healthier foods!

At the two-week point, I began to add one inflammatory food back into my diet. I chose wheat. I waited a few days to start feeling badly, but I felt fine. However, after a week, I noticed that my joints were achy. I went back to the original simple diet for two weeks, then added dairy. I found out within a few minutes where my runny nose came from.

During this time, I kept a food diary. It was helpful to see what foods caused discomfort and what foods were fine for me to eat. I would recommend trying a two-week elimination diet, especially if you often experience headaches, stomach aches, skin problems, sinus problems, and bloating. After two weeks, reintroduce just one common inflammatory item. Continue on the elimination diet while consuming the one potential inflammatory item. If you have no adverse symptoms, it should be fine for you to ingest on a regular basis. If you do have discomfort or feel ill while eating the potentially inflammatory food, perhaps you'd do best to avoid it.

In the appendix, you'll find a sample elimination diet plan.

Bottom Line

Food is nourishment and fuel for our bodies. I think there should also be enjoyment in eating. Perhaps you'll do well on the 40/40/20 split, or you may do better with lower carbohydrate and higher fats. The takeaway is that as long as your daily caloric intake is moderate, and you're staying active, almost any meal plan will be effective. Find the ones that are sustainable and moderately enjoyable. Most importantly, be sure that it is one that gives you the energy needed to conquer your goals!

Dieting and the Pendulum

The Pendulum

Whether it's for a fitness competition, a special event, or for a personal resolution, we have all dieted at some point. After the diet, there is usually a rebound. This can lead to weight gain, and increases the likelihood of fat gain. When we restrict calories for a long time, we end up eating foods that are high-fat and/or high-sugar. Our bodies don't know that we've been dieting; instead it operates as if we were starving. Excess calories are easily shuttled to fat cells because the body doesn't know when it will have enough calories again, so it stores as much as possible. This creates a pendulum effect. The harder and longer we diet, the more extreme the swing will be once we stop dieting. Also, the more times we go through phases of dieting and rebound, the more likely we are to continue to hold stubborn fat. Once we're aware of this, we're better able to keep the pendulum balanced in the middle. The first step, even if you're looking to lean down, is to stop dieting. In this chapter, we'll look at the effects of dieting, and how to work with your body and mind to achieve lasting results.

DIEt

What comes to mind when you think of the word "diet?" For many of us, it means counting calories, restrictions, and a temporary fix. A diet is almost impossible to maintain on a long-term basis. To understand why, we must look at how our bodies and minds work. Traditional dieting relies heavily on our willpower – the restriction of calories is maintained by our motivation and discipline. But, when restrictions are placed upon us, we automatically think in terms of scarcity and feel the effects of it. Thoughts of scarcity can cause us to crave the foods we're not allowed to have. Creating a long-term caloric deficit can cause our bodies to crave high-calorie, nutrient-dense food. This is a survival mechanism, created long ago when we'd have to go periods of time without food. Though we have evolved in many ways, this instinct for survival is hard wired in all of us.

So, we have unknowingly set up a scenario where we pit willpower against instinct. Ultimately, instinct prevails. We usually eat foods we wouldn't normally choose... and in mass quantities.

Perhaps the best example of this is the Minnesota Semi-Starvation experiment conducted from 1944-45 by University of Minnesota physiologist Ancel Keys. 36 men volunteered for the year-long study. They spent 3 months consuming 3,200 calories, 6 months consuming 1,600 calories, and 3 months in recovery from the semi-starvation. During the experiment, the men obsessed over food. Some made scrap books of food pictures, some tried to eat from the garbage, and one man tried to eat his shoe. They became lethargic, their skin grew dull and rough, and some lost hair. After the study, many gained back the weight they had lost, plus 10% more. Two had to be admitted for psychiatric care. It was a ground-breaking experiment. Though it was done to an extreme, it shows how detrimental dieting can be.

Eating Less but Weighing More

The Minnesota Semi-Starvation Experiment showed that an ongoing caloric deficit can have lasting effects. Another point to consider is how the body is so amazingly adaptive that it will conserve calories in other ways we might not realize. We'll experience a decrease in non-exercise activity thermogenesis (NEAT).

NEAT is the amount of calories we expend just by walking around, doing chores, etc. In addition to our basal metabolic rate, we can burn an additional 600-1,000 calories just by being active. When we're eating enough, we tend to move around more. But when calories are decreased, the body adjusts by becoming less active. The combination of decreased calories and decreased activity levels can lead to a plateau in progress, or even lead to weight gain. Workout intensity usually suffers, too. Or, we'll have just enough energy to complete a workout, only to veg out on the couch for the rest of the night.

A simple fix is to make sure calories never drop below the basal metabolic rate (BMR), and to eat frequent, balanced meals. If you're training or have a career that keeps you moving, it's a good idea to add calories to your BMR caloric intake.

Later, Single-serve, and Conditioning

A great way to make progress while enjoying food is to not label anything "off-limits." That being said, I think it's important to have some strategies when it comes to cravings. I have split three strategies I employ: "later," "single-serve," and "post-cheat feeling conditioning."

If I'm craving something during the week, I tell myself I can have it "later." Usually the thought fades in 15 minutes and I forget all about the craving. In order to create balance in life, we must study how the body and mind work. We want what we can't have, and we want more when we feel deprived. Knowing that I can eat drive-thru food if I want to makes it a lot less appealing (if that was even possible).

Sometimes the craving lingers, and I don't want to wait until "later" to have something. In this case, I'll buy a single-serve of whatever it is that I'm set on. A couple of squares of dark chocolate, a small ice cream, or a packet of peanut butter on an apple all makes delicious, sweet-tooth-taming treats. Single-serve items also keep entire boxes of potential "trigger foods" out of the cupboard.

Another way to avoid overeating on unhealthy foods is to imagine how you feel after you've eaten them. I love pizza, and could eat an entire pie... but I feel awful afterward. I have a stomach ache, headache, bloating, and I feel sluggish. If I want to overindulge, I vividly recreate those feelings I have after I've eaten too much. I then decide if it's worth it. Most of the time, it's not. But, sometimes it is. I enjoy every bite. Meals are much more enjoyable when we're in control and when we make the choices!

Trigger Foods

I think we all have certain trigger foods. Once these are recognized, it's a good idea to keep them away from easy reach. The easiest way to not go on a peanut butter bender is to not have it within easy reach. Do you know what foods cause you to ignore your off switch? I know that I can't have peanut butter, rice cakes, or chocolate in my house. The old adage, "out of sight, out of mind", comes into play here.

If you have kids or work in situations where you can't avoid trigger foods, this can be challenging. Some creativity is necessary. Once you have identified the trigger foods, think of replacement foods that are less appealing. This can be as easy as switching from creamy peanut butter to chunky peanut butter. Also, remember that there is no food in this world that you can't have – you just choose not to partake.

Try a Treat Meal

Treat meals can be a great way to indulge without going overboard. This can help cut cravings and give you something to look forward to. I have always enjoyed going out for sushi, a steak and potato, or ice cream after a Saturday leg workout. Two keys to a successful treat meal are planning in advance, and ending the splurge as soon as the meal is over. Think about what you might be craving during the week, and set parameters before indulging. If the meal is a steak and potato, decide what cut of steak, portion size, and other sides. It might be tempting to order dessert, but remember you can have it next time. When your meal arrives, be mindful and present. Savor each bite, and take your time to enjoy the meal.

What happens if you give in and eat a dessert? You'll be ok. You can use the additional calories as fuel in the gym. Try not to be hard on yourself, and use self-talk to move on without lamenting over the extra calories.

Don't Sweat the Small Stuff

I think it's important to weigh foods when embarking on the lifestyle change. But don't stress about exact portions. When we eat the same foods at the same time every day, our bodies get accustomed and comfortable with the plan. When we're comfortable, we tend to plateau. This is why under-eating, over-eating, and occasionally skipping a meal might help keep our metabolisms revved.

Sometimes, when we weigh foods, we become fixated on exact proportions. It can make eating out or enjoying food very difficult. So, weigh foods until you have a handle on how much a portion size is, and then feel free to push the scale aside.

Be Leery of Labels

I think we have all found ourselves eating according to certain labels. Some examples are "fat free," "low carb," or "Paleo." By eliminating entire food groups (barring allergies), we have effectively labeled these foods "off-limits." A quick search of "Paleo bread recipes" will show just how much those on that diet crave bread. Many of the processed/boxed foods that are geared toward labels are essentially junk food. They're often loaded with added sugar, fat, preservatives, and fillers. If you can, allow all foods in moderation, and make simple, one-ingredient food choices. Some examples include chicken, eggs, fish, oats, rice, apples, bananas, spinach, squash, sweet potatoes, and broccoli. At the grocery store, try to do most of your shopping around the perimeter of the store. There you'll find the produce, seafood, butcher, and dairy sections. Tempting junk food is often placed at eye-level on the end caps and at the register. Make a list of items you need before you shop. Also, try not to shop when hungry. We're more apt to impulse buy items we don't need when we're hungry or when we're aimlessly browsing.

The Miracle Pill

We don't fall for "get rich quick" schemes; so it's a wonder so many of us fall for "get fit quick" schemes! Juices, pills, shots, and apparel flood the media. Their promises are glossier than their packaging. The thought of getting to a goal faster is alluring, but it's also unlikely. Many fads will provide short-term results, but just like a diet, it is temporary. One of the best ways to make a big change is to make a series of small changes over time. Being fit and healthy can be a lifestyle – it can be your lifestyle! Some examples of small changes are to reduce sugary drinks, cook more meals rather than having fast food, and gradually increasing your activity level.

Our metabolisms are elastic. Drastic, long-term caloric deprivation will slow it down, but it will increase with time. It's just going to depend on your body and your ability to be patient in bringing yourself back to equilibrium. Give yourself time to make this transition. You may gain a few pounds in the short term, but know that your long term goals can be achieved and sustained when you've stopped the pendulum swing.

Visualization, Materialization, and Motivation

You're the Star

Imagine your perfect life. Imagine it in detail: the house you live in, the people around you, and what you do on a daily basis. Now, imagine your perfect physique: your curves, your strength, and how you move. Can you see your life in perfect detail? How does it compare to your life at this very moment?

Before you can achieve anything, you must have a clear mental image of it. In this chapter, we'll go over how to visualize, create motivation, protect your energy, and materialize the wishes of your heart. By carefully deciding what you really want, you're creating a blueprint for following your passion. This may take some time, and that's ok. Don't rush into developing your goals. I often think that we have our true desires mixed with the "shoulds." We might want to train for a competition, but think we "should" be training to fit into a certain pant size.

Often, when we try to live up to others' expectations, we end up pleasing no one. You get to write your own story. You are the star of your show. No matter how silly the goal is, write it down. I keep separate lists – one for physique and athletic goals, one for career, and one for the fun things I want in my life just because I want them.

See It in Perfect Detail

In early 2010, I set a goal to win the Ms. Figure Olympia. I shared my goal with a few people. Each one said that I was crazy to think that I could win the biggest contest in bodybuilding after my rookie season. I didn't listen to the opinions. Right before bed, I would play out the prejudging and the night show – down to the smallest detail. I could see the sweep of my quads, the width of my lats, each step on stage, and each pose. I could feel the cold air of the arena and the hot lights at the night show. Each night, I'd imagine the finals and the awards presentation. I'd see other competitors walk to center stage for their awards. I felt the excitement as I waited for my name to be called. I could hear the emcee announce 2nd place, and felt a warm hug from the girl next to me. I won... I won!

The visualization became so real to me that I could feel the weight of the trophy in my hands. I trained and prepared like I had already won. When it came time to for the award ceremony in Las Vegas, I had a surprised look on my face when my name was announced as the winner. The crazy thing is... I wasn't as surprised that I won as I was surprised that it happened exactly the way I imagined it would.

First, Train with your Brain

It might seem like a strange notion, but consider this for a moment: you begin your workout with a goal to lift your bodyweight for reps. You visualize yourself going through the exercise successfully as you're warming up. The picture you have created in your head is vivid, and you have imagined the smallest details. You performed the lift exactly how you rehearsed it in your head. The challenging set is a success! You'll probably leave the gym with a little more confidence and the knowledge that you can achieve the things you set your mind to. With the same visualization process, imagine one of your non-fitness goals. See yourself having or doing exactly what you wish to do. Imagine the details of your greatest goal. Strive toward that goal with the confidence you have found while pushing yourself at the gym.

I truly believe that if you focus on something, with all of the good energy you have, it will be yours. Can you recall a time when you wanted something so badly that it was all you could think about? Did you get it, do it, or accomplish it? I'll bet the answer to both of those questions is "yes!" Everything that exists in our lives has been brought about by us.

Success Starts with the Mind

In his book, *As A Man Thinketh*, James Allen writes "good thoughts and actions can never in the long run produce bad results." We are a combination of the thoughts we focus on. When we look to the world as full of opportunities and visualize our success, success must come.

In another section, Allen writes, "nothing can come from corn, but corn. Nothing can come from nettles, but nettles. Men understand this law in the natural world and work with it. But few understand it in the mental and moral world, though its operation there is just as simple and undeviating." Many of us tend to focus on negative parts of our lives, and focus on the things we absolutely do not want to do. When we do this, we place energy and effort on these things - unknowingly drawing them closer and making them stronger. It's important, especially just starting out, to become aware of our thoughts.

Negative thoughts can become a habit, and rerouting our thoughts is the first step to positive visualization. The next step is replacing the old negative thoughts with the clearly defined goals and thoughts of our success.

An analogy that I have always loved is comparing our thoughts and mind to a field. What we plant in the field will grow, and what thoughts we plant in our minds will grow. What we choose to water in the field will grow faster, and the thoughts we focus on will grow faster. We can put our energy towards weeds, or bad thoughts. Or, we can put our energy towards beautiful flowers, or good thoughts. What is growing in your field? What thoughts are you watering with your energy? With practice, it becomes easier to focus on the positive aspects of life and create an environment that favors success.

Visualize to Materialize

Very often, the thing that slows us down is not the lack of resources or time – it's the aimless drifting and vague goals. In order to accomplish something, we must decide and define our objectives. There aren't enough parameters in the fuzzy goal of wanting to "lose weight." Think about the details of the physique you want. By creating a perfect mental image and keeping attention on that image, it begins to materialize. But there is no materialization without visualization.

Take a few moments to set and prioritize goals. You might want to focus on one main project, or it may be a list of 3-4 smaller achievements. Write them down, along with every detail you can imagine. I think that the universe has a way of sending us what we ask for, but we may receive it in ways we don't like if we don't ask in perfect detail.

For example, I set a goal to travel more. I didn't specify how I wanted to travel, just that I wanted to see the world. Shortly after I put my energy on the goal, I received a request to do more international appearances. But instead of traveling in comfort, my flights had many connections and I often wouldn't have my itinerary until hours before I was supposed to leave. I had to pay for many things out of pocket and often worried about my safety. Yes, I got what I wanted – more travel; but I learned to specify my wishes in greater detail after that experience. Know exactly what you want and set your energy upon achieving it.

Can You Do It?

Make sure you can realistically devote enough time, attention, and energy to start and maintain progress. Simply wishing for a change won't bring it. I think we need lofty goals. A challenge and a stretch will bring change. However, stretch too far and it's easy to wear yourself thin. Can you do it? Yes, you can – 100%!

Once you have clearly defined goals, protect them dearly. People will criticize and plant seeds of doubt – don't let these seeds take root. Be careful of your thoughts, too. Your dreams are sacred, and your mind is your kingdom. Change is a scary thing. Fear tends to creep in and paralyze. Know that it's normal to have your own doubts and fears. Yet, also know that your ability and resolve is strong enough to help you achieve anything you set your mind to.

Just like repetition in the weight room brings about nicely shaped muscles; repetition of positive thoughts and goals bring about a beautiful mind – and success!

Motivation

Truly lasting motivation and drive is intrinsic, meaning it is derived from within. What do you really want? Dig deep, and do some soul-searching. When it comes to fitness goals, many of us have goals to trim down or lose weight. Setting a goal based in self-judgment makes it difficult to accomplish. This is not a goal that comes from the heart. It's almost as if you're beating yourself down before you even begin. Your goal doesn't have to be fitness-based. Perhaps you'd like to become a proficient public speaker, save money to travel the world, or buy a house. Developing an athlete's mindset, improving perspective, and adding structure through fitness will help you achieve goals that stretch beyond fitness.

Motivation also comes from a sense of purpose. Yet it's not simply enough to seek an outer purpose. Certainly, we all want a better job, a nice car, to win competitions, and to have great relationships. As hard as we strive, these goals can't provide lasting happiness because they're often tied to variables beyond our control. Lasting motivation and greater happiness is derived from a distinct inner purpose. What does this mean, exactly? Your inner purpose is your very core: your thoughts, outlook, perception, and mindset. It's about appreciating today – not waiting to be happy when you fit into your jeans or run your goal 5k time.

 The joy is in the journey. Whether we know it or not, we can choose how we wish to perceive ourselves and our life in general. Why not choose to see our strengths, blessings, and opportunities?

Lasting motivation can be attained by connecting with your passion. Think about the things that you enjoy doing. I think it would be tough to deny that we all have an outer motivation to improve looks, but I've found that the inner motivation can often help us achieve the outer purpose without much additional effort. For example, a passion for biking will lead to toned legs, or swimming can help to achieve that lean look. Fitness related goals are more easily attained when the activity is truly enjoyable.

The Little Critic

On the road to establishing goals and sparking motivation, the little critic's voice inside us will point us to what we want. But, it will also whisper (or shout) its doubts and fears. When we're following a goal that we want more than anything, our efforts will be stronger than our fears if we have faith in our ability to achieve our goals. Know that this self-doubt and fear is normal and part of the process. Some common doubts and fears include:

- I'm too old
- It will take too much time
- People will think I'm crazy
- I don't have enough knowledge
- I'm not talented enough
- What if....?

Even the bravest of the brave have self-defeating thoughts. Knowing this makes us stronger. Be ready to confront that wimpy voice. It's the only thing that stands in the way of your success. Don't let the little critic come between you and your greatness.

Positive affirmations can go a long way in bolstering motivation. When our doubts and fears creep in, be aware of them. Don't add fuel to the fire by entertaining the negative thoughts. Instead, try replacing them with some of these affirmations:

- I am strong enough
- I am capable
- I will achieve _____
- I am smart enough
- I am courageous

- I like myself

At this point, you might think I'm nuts. But, try it. Choose a phrase and repeat it 10-20 times when a negative thought comes up. You'll find that it will strengthen your resolve. To understand why this works, we take a look at our minds — conscious and subconscious.

Appendix

Here are some of the workouts I have used in the last few years. The "building" workouts will be higher volume (4-5 sets), while the "get lean" workouts will have more circuits and supersets. These can be used as a template to help you design your own training split, or you can follow them to get a feel for the different training styles.

I also wanted to include a sample guide for an elimination meal plan. This can be used to cut out potentially inflammatory foods. There's also a sample 40/40/20 meal guide. These can both be expanded by substituting like foods. Some easy guidelines:

- Carbohydrates are pretty much interchangeable: quinoa, pumpkin, rice cakes, sweet potato, rice, or squash can all work well. Also, veggie portions (leafy greens are considered a "free food," if you want to eat a whole bag of fresh spinach..go for it.
- Meat substitutions: tuna steak, venison, chicken breast, lean ground turkey, tilapia, orange roughy, and egg whites are all great.
- Condiments: salsa, mustard, low-fat/low-sugar dressing, no sugar added ketchup, sugar free syrup, all seasonings, and can use a small amount of olive oil in cooking. Try different spices for flavor without added calories.
- If you think you're going to miss a meal, have a protein shake. It's very important to eat every few hours.

Sample 3x Week Building Program:

<u>Monday – Legs (1 min between sets)</u>

- Single-leg leg press, knee to chest, 5x8 each leg
- Straight leg deadlift, 4x10
- Leg extension, 4x10
- Leg curls, 4x10
- Standing calf raise, 4x10

<u>Tuesday – Off</u>

<u>Wednesday – Shoulders and Arms</u>

- Dumbbell shoulder press or military press, 4x10
- Rear delts raises on incline bench (stomach-down) with dumbbells, 4x10
- One-arm dumbbell lateral raise, body at a 45 degree angle, 4x10 each arm
- Weighted bench dips, 4x10
- Drag curls with EZ bar, 4x10
- Triceps kickback with rope, 4x8
- Standing biceps curls with rope on cable. 4x8

<u>Thursday – Off</u>

<u>Friday – Back and Chest</u>

- Wide-grip lat pull down, hold mid-rep, 4x10
- Incline bench, 4x8
- EZ pullovers with dumbbell on flat bench, 4x8
- Incline dumbbell flyes, 4x8
- Bent-over single arm dumbbell rows, 4x8 each side
- Decline cable flyes, 4x8

Sample 5x Week Building Program:

<u>Monday –Shoulders (1 minute-1:30 rest between sets)</u>

- Dumbbell shoulder press or military press, 5x8
- Upright rows on cable, 5x8
- Dumbbell seated front raise, 5x8
- Dumbbell rear delts raise, stomach-down on incline bench, 5x8
- Dumbbell standing single-arm lateral raise, body at 45 degree angle, 5x8

<u>Tuesday –Legs (1minute-1:30 rest between sets)</u>

- Back squats, pause at the bottom of the rep for 2 seconds, 5x8
- Standing calf raise, 5x8
- Straight leg deadlift, 5x8
- Weighted bridge, 3x15
- Leg extensions, 5x8
- Leg curl, 5x8
- Seated calf raise, 3x20

<u>Wednesday – Arms (1minute -1:30 rest between sets)</u>

- Plank chin-ups on Smith machine, 3x as many as you can do
- Weighted bench dips, 5x8
- Drag curls, 5x8
- Skullcrushers on bench, 5x8
- Cable double biceps curls, 5x8
- Cable rope push downs, 5x8

<u>Thursday – Back (1minute-1:30 rest between sets)</u>

- T-bar rows, 5x8
- Dumbbell bent over single-arm rows, 5x8 each side

- Wide-grip lat pull down, pause 2 seconds mid-rep), 5x8
- Cable rope high pulls, 5x8
- Dumbbell EZ pullovers on bench, 5x8
- Close-grip lat pull down, 5x8

Friday – Chest (1 minute-1:30 rest between sets)

- Incline bench, pause mid-rep, 5x8
- Cable incline flyes, 4x10
- Push ups, 3x as many as you can do
- Cable flat flyes, 4x10
- Decline push ups, feet up on bench, 3x10
- Dips, body weight leaning forward, 3x as many as you can do

Sample 4-5x Week Push-Pull Workout:

Monday – Back/Chest (30-45 seconds rest between sets)

- Bent over barbell rows, 4x8
- Single-arm incline bench, 4x8 each arm
- Dumbbell incline flyes, 3x12, superset with dumbbell incline rows, stomach-down on bench, 3x12
- Wide-grip lat pull down, 3x12, superset with push-ups, 3x15
- Dumbbell alternating single-arm bench, 3x8 each arm, superset with dumbbell EZ pullovers, 3x12

Tuesday – Legs/Glutes (45 seconds rest between sets)

- Front squats, 4x10
- RDL's, 4x10
- Hack squats, 3x15
- Lying leg curl, 4x8, superset with hip thrusts, 4x12
- Standing calf raise, 3x12, superset with hip abductor, 3x15

<u>Wednesday – Off or HIIT/Conditioning/Cardio</u>

- See following pages for workouts

<u>Thursday – Shoulders/Arms (30-45 seconds between sets)</u>

- Military press, 4x10, or push press
- T-bar rows, 4x10
- Arnold press, 3x15
- Giant set on cable with rope attachment, 3x10 – upright rows, overhead triceps extension, rope curls, diamond push ups
- Dumbbell hammer curls, 3x12, superset with dumbbell triceps kick backs, 3x12

<u>Friday – Plyos and Legs (1 minute between sets)</u>

- Optional hang snatch warm up, 3x3
- 10 reps each of speed squats, dynamic step-ups, line jumps, rocket jumps
- Goblet squats, 3x15
- Leg extensions, 3x12, superset with single-leg hip thrusts
- Cable rope pull throughs, 3x10, superset with seated leg curl, 3x10
- Seated calf raise, 3x15, superset with glute bridges, 3x20

Sample 4-5x Week Get Lean Supersets Workout:

<u>Monday – Back/Shoulders/Abs (45 seconds rest between sets)</u>

- T-bar rows, superset with dumbbell standing shoulder press, 3x15
- Wide-grip lat pull down with dumbbell upright rows, 3x15, plank 30 seconds after each superset (straight, then right and left side)

- Close-grip cable rows with seated dumbbell lateral raise, 3x15, with 30 v-ups
- Single-arm cable pull downs (stabilize yourself in a lunge position- one knee on the ground) with standing cable front raise, 3x15, with 30 crunches

Tuesday – Legs/Plyos (1 minute between sets)

Warm up plyo circuit – go through once and do 10 reps per exercise:
- Box or bench jumps
- 180 degree jumps
- Depth jumps
- Tuck jumps

- Back squats to parallel with standing calf raise, 3x15
- Straight leg deadlift with walking lunges, 3x12
- Leg curl with leg extension, 3x15

Wednesday – Cardio or Off

Thursday – Chest/Arms (1 minute recovery between sets)

- EZ bar on flat bench – bench press, skullcrushers, drag curls (standing with EZ bar), 3x15
- Dumbbell incline bench press, close grip push ups, hammer curls (seated on incline), 3x15
- On cable machine – standing incline flyes, cable push downs (with rope), with rope cable curls, 3x15
- 3x20 push ups

Friday – Legs (45 seconds between sets)

- Weighted step ups – 3x8 each leg, alternating legs

- Front squats with standing calf raise (holding dumbbells), 3x15
- Bulgarian split squats with single-leg straight-leg deadlifts, 3x12 each leg
- Weighted walking lunges, 3x12 each leg

Sample Sprints and Conditioning Workouts

<u>At The Track</u>

- Sprint the straight-a-ways, walk the curves, 12 sprints total
- 10x50M accelerations. 3-5 minutes between sprints
- 6x150M, 3-5 minutes between sprints
- 500/400/300M, 4 minutes rest between sprints
- 4x200M, 4-5 minutes between sprints
- 14 diagonals – stride diagonals on the field, walk the short side of the field for recovery between strides

<u>At the Gym</u>

- Kettlebell/medicine ball tabata : 20 seconds of kettlebell swings, 10 seconds rest, 20 seconds of medicine ball slams, 10 seconds rest, 20 seconds of jumping rope, 10 seconds rest, 20 seconds of clap jacks, 10 seconds rest. Repeat once. Cool down
- Barbell complex - between 5-10 reps per exercise, no breaks: hang cleans, push jerks, overhead squats, bent over rows, straight leg deadlifts
- Tabata on cardio equipment: 8x20 seconds all out, 10 seconds rest, on the machine of your choice

Sample Meals

This is a simple guide, based on the foods I would normally eat. Feel free to adjust, add, or otherwise modify these suggestions.

40/40/20 Meal Guide

- 4 egg whites, one egg, with 1/2c oats
- Protein shake, medium apple (this meal can be moved to post-workout)
- 4oz chicken, 6oz sweet potato, spinach salad
- 4 oz chicken, 1/2c cooked brown rice
- 4-6oz steak, steamed veggies
- Optional snack – 5 egg white omelet or 2 eggs

Sample Elimination Meal Guide

- 5 egg whites, 1/4c buckwheat (measured dry)
- 4oz chicken, 1/2c cooked brown rice, spinach salad with splash of oil and vinegar
- 4oz chicken, one medium apple
- 4oz lean beef or salmon, 1/2 avocado, steamed veggies
- 2 eggs

Works Cited

Rolls, Barbara J. *The Volumetrics Eating Plan: Techniques and Recipes for Feeling Full on Fewer Calories*. New York: Harper, 2007. Print.

"Journal of Nutrition." *They Starved So That Others Be Better Fed: Remembering Ancel Keys and the Minnesota Experiment*. Web. 26 Mar. 2015.
<http://jn.nutrition.org/content/135/6/1347.full>.

Muscolino, Joseph E. *Kinesiology: The Skeletal System and Muscle Function*. 2nd ed. St. Louis, Mo.: Mosby/Elsevier, 2011. Print.

"BMI Calculator." *BMR Calculator*. Web. 26 Mar. 2015.
<http://www.bmi-calculator.net/bmr-calculator/>.

About

Erin is a former 2x Ms Figure Olympia and Junior All-American track athlete. Her love for training started at a very young age while running alongside her horses. She earned an academic scholarship to attend the University of Florida, and was invited to walk on the varsity track team. Once on the team, she earned an athletic scholarship and Jr. All-American status in the high jump. She was the first Lady Gator to compete in the indoor pentathlon. After college, she missed the Olympic Qualifying Standard by 3cm with a jump of 5'11". This prompted her to try figure competitions. She earned Pro status by winning the Overall Figure Championship at the 2008 NPC Nationals. In 2010, she won her first Figure Olympia Champion title. Between 2008 and 2010, she overcame various roadblocks and hardships to win the biggest contest in bodybuilding. She accomplished this with no coach or trainer, and as a lifetime natural athlete.

She currently speaks to high school athletes about priorities, goal-setting, visualization, and mindset. In addition to speaking, she runs seminars geared toward training, living a healthy lifestyle, and improving self-esteem.

"I am motivated to be better than my previous best," she says. "I'm also motivated by the people I meet along the way. It's just a big fitness family, and to be able to inspire and motivate others keeps me going. Ultimately, I want to teach people how to find their own unique greatness. I also want to show them that success in the gym translates to confidence and success in all other aspects of life."

EDUCATION
UNIVERSITY OF FLORIDA, Warrington College of Business
Master of Science Coursework in Business Management
UNIVERSITY OF FLORIDA, College of Natural Resources and Environment
Bachelor of Arts in Environmental Science - Environmental Policy, December 2002
AMFPT Certified Personal Trainer

SKILLS

Published Author

Created a comprehensive 28-day training/diet plan for Bodybuilding.com

Created content for Muscle & Fitness Hers "Road to Olympia" training videos

Ran a series of seminars and training camps in major Australian cities

Created F.A.S.T. and 20/20 training techniques

Regularly speak for groups, from high school athletes to weekend athletes

Studied at Patel Conservatory for acting on camera, football sideline radio reporter

Online Fitness Coach and Consultant

Toastmaster

ACHIEVEMENTS

2X Ms. Figure Olympia Champion

Arnold Classic Figure Champion

12 IFBB Figure Titles

Lifetime Natural Athlete

Former Junior All-American High Jumper and Heptathlete

Current USATF Athlete

COVERS

Oxygen Magazine Australia – March 2015

Oxygen Magazine –September 2014

Oxygen Magazine - December 2013

Jupiter Magazine – March, 2013

Muscle & Fitness Hers –February 2013

Oxygen Magazine - February 2012

Oxygen Magazine –July 2010

Healthy Living Magazine - July 2011

Muscle & Body Magazine - September 2011

Ocala Magazine - October 2011

Connect With Me!

Website: www.erinstern.com
YouTube: www.youtube.com/erinstern5
Facebook: www.facebook.com/erinstern
            www.facebook.com/fiterin
Twitter: www.twitter.com/erinfast
Instagram: www.instagram.com/erinstern5

A big thanks to Jonathan Milton for editing this book! Contact him for editing and freelance writing services at www.jonathanmilton.net.

Made in the USA
Monee, IL
22 July 2020